Kids Thrive at Every Size

How to Nourish Your Big, Small, or In-Between
Child for a Lifetime of Health and Happiness

Jill Castle, MS, RD

Foreword by Jessica Dudley, MD

WORKMAN PUBLISHING • NEW YORK

Workman
Workman Publishing
Hachette Book Group, Inc.
1290 Avenue of the Americas
New York, NY 10104
workman.com

Workman is an imprint of Workman Publishing, a division of Hachette Book Group, Inc. The Workman name and logo are registered trademarks of Hachette Book Group, Inc.

Design by Galen Smith

The publisher is not responsible for websites (or their content) that are not owned by the publisher.

Workman books may be purchased in bulk for business, educational, or promotional use. For information, please contact your local bookseller or the Hachette Book Group Special Markets Department at special.markets@hbgusa.com.

Disclaimer Note:

This book is intended to be a resource and guide for those wishing to know how to instill healthful lifestyle habits in young children. The information in this book is based on evidence, experience, and the expertise of others in their respective fields. It is not intended to replace treatment from a health-care provider or your medical or psychological team. The information presented in this book is general. Specific medical advice should be tailored to your individual child with your health-care provider. The stories and quotes in this book come from real people, or a composite of real experiences from the author's work. Names and identifying details have been changed to protect their privacy.

Library of Congress Cataloging-in-Publication Data is available.

ISBN 978-1-5235-2183-8 (paperback)

First Edition August 2024

Printed in China on responsibly sourced paper.

10 9 8 7 6 5 4 3 2 1

For my "Family Castle"

You're the best thing that has ever happened to me.

CONTENTS

FOREWORD

by Jessica Dudley, MD

ppearance. Weight. Health. Diet. Exercise. These are things that many of us (most of us) think about daily.

As a former practicing physician, it was my job to think about them. Like so many of us, my patients struggled with the everyday challenges of getting regular exercise and eating a balanced diet or wrestling with weight that may have been impacting their physical or emotional well-being. Over the years, I'd try different approaches to counseling around health, weight, diet, and exercise. In some cases, my patients made a shift or change which led to improved health and emotional outcomes, but for the overwhelming majority the struggle continued.

As a parent to three young children (now grown), it also felt like it was my job to think about health, diet, and exercise. I encouraged my kids to eat healthy foods; I tried to make sure we ate together as a family even when they were very little; and we were always very active. But the job wasn't as straightforward as I thought it would be. One of my kids always seemed hungrier and ate faster and more voraciously. I worried about her and became focused on her physical well-being. I restricted sweets in our home and monitored her eating habits. I got her a Fitbit, which she diligently wore, and then later I found her a personal trainer to help her with exercise. I thought I was helping. Then, one day, she revealed to me that she dreaded going to the personal trainer—the visits made her anxious and she begged me to not make her go. That's when I realized that my efforts had been harming my child, not helping her.

My child is now an adult on her own journey. If I had read *Kids Thrive at Every Size* twenty years ago, I believe I would have been a better partner and advocate for her when she was young. I would have been more of a listener and supporter and less of a fixer and a solver. I would have understood that health isn't just appearance and weight, diet, and exercise, but far more comprehensive and holistic. I would have learned that as parents, our job is to help our children develop their own positive approach to health and wellness. And to do this requires a whole-child approach—one that centers their emotional well-being alongside their physical health.

If this seems like an overwhelming task, fear not. With this book, Jill Castle provides a road map for parents, one that connects health across disciplines—physical, emotional, and behavioral. She shows us that raising kids who are healthy and physically and emotionally well starts with the family. It is not a game that you win or lose, but one that evolves as you move forward, stay positive, and keep learning.

As I read Jill's book, I thought about the many things I wished I had done differently. But as I read on, I realized that this is not about "right or wrong," but instead a learning journey . . . and I have learned a lot along the way. Jill's book helped pull so many of my experiences into a clear focus and left me feeling empowered and optimistic.

I've read countless books on parenting, but never one quite like this. *Kids Thrive at Every Size* guides parents forward with supportive, actionable habits while centering on both physical health and emotional well-being.

The impossible exists only until we find a way to make it possible.

—MIKE HORN

· ·

INTRODUCTION

· ·

So, what prompted you to pick up this book? Maybe your child is a bigger kid, and you're worried about their size and eating habits. Or your child loves sweets, sneaks food, and can't seem to stop eating . . . and this scares you. Perhaps you have a family history of heart disease or diabetes, or you grew up with a larger body yourself. Maybe your kid is smaller in size, struggles with picky eating, or there's a family history of an eating disorder. You're keen on preventing history from repeating itself. Possibly, your child was bullied about their size or is asking questions you're not sure how to answer. More likely, though, you're in the thick of parenting, want to do right by your child, and picked up this book as your guide to establishing good habits.

I'm glad we've found each other! If you are worried, suspect you're on the wrong path, or don't have a path at all, you're absolutely in the right place. Because without a road map for healthful lifestyle behaviors, chances are good you'll face challenges down the road. And for those of you asking, *What is the right path?* I hear you.

"Peter's the biggest kid in his second-grade class. He's always been a big boy, but he's started to notice he's bigger than the other kids," said Ann, mom of eight-year-old Peter. "I think he's getting comments about his weight at school. He hasn't mentioned it—but I have a hunch." Ann worried that Peter's self-esteem was suffering. She wanted help—the "right" kind of help that would encourage his health and protect his self-esteem. Parents of children who are smaller, like Shelly, are equally concerned about their kid's self-esteem, growth, and health. "My five-year-old Max has always been small and is barely on the growth curve," Shelly said. "I worry about him starting school, not eating enough during the day, and getting teased for his size."

Kids come in all shapes and sizes. Today more families are raising kids with larger bodies than at any other point in our history. At the other end of the spectrum are kids who have smaller bodies. And then there are those in between. No matter your child's size, you may fret about the habits they're developing, and whether they're happy and secure. The instinct to protect your child, whether they're larger, smaller, or in-between, is universal and totally appropriate, especially today.

Kids are growing up in a world that values what they look like above almost everything else. As an extension, unfortunately, your child's health may be summed up based on their size or appearance. If they're larger, they're presumed to be eating too much, choosing the wrong foods, or neglecting a healthy habit like exercise. Yes, some children do exceed their nutritional needs and live a sedentary lifestyle, but it is also true that size is genetically inherited and larger children can be healthy and free from health concerns. The size of a child does not predict their health.

If a child is smaller, you may get questions about whether they're getting enough nutrition, are ill, or have an eating disorder. True, some children may have ongoing challenges that affect their size and stature, such as a history of premature birth, picky eating, food allergies, or another chronic health condition. Or they may experience food insecurity, which may prevent them from getting enough consistently available nutritious food. But many children who are smaller are genetically inclined to be so.

The most dangerous assumption we make is about kids who are not small or large, but in-between. We think they're healthy simply because of their size. But kids who are midsize aren't necessarily as healthy as they appear. They may have nutrient inadequacies, unhealthy eating habits, and lifestyle behaviors that gamble their future health. One only has to look at the eating and lifestyle behaviors of all children in the United States to know they're facing an uncertain future. Many children eat too many nutrient-poor foods, don't get enough sleep, and fall short of their age-appropriate physical activity goals.

> **#TruthBomb:**
> Children of all shapes and sizes can be healthy. Don't assume a child's size, shape, or appearance is a marker for ill health.

Adding to health concerns is what *every* parent of *every* child is worried about today: the struggle with self-esteem and mental health. Increasingly, children of *every* size are experiencing mental health concerns. According to the Centers for Disease Control and Prevention (CDC), prior to the COVID-19 pandemic about 7 percent of children and teens had anxiety, and 3 percent had depression. However, during and after, rates dramatically increased with generalized anxiety at a prevalence of 20 percent and depression at 25 percent in school-age children. And the latest statistics from the CDC suggest that "teens girls and teens who identify as lesbian, gay, bisexual, and questioning (LGBQ+) are experiencing extremely high levels of mental distress, violence, and substance use." We're seeing the highest rates of sadness, violence, and hopelessness ever reported. If your child has a larger or smaller body, you may be very concerned about their mental well-being.

Societal norms and biases about appearance may disturb a child's body image. Children as young as three show dissatisfaction with their bodies, and girls and boys as young as six wish they were thinner. By middle school, half of all girls and a third of all boys want a thinner body. Girls diet to lose weight, obsessively exercise, and sometimes develop an eating disorder along the way. Seventy-five percent of teen boys are unhappy with their bodies and want to be bigger and more muscular. "Bigorexia," a new term for boys who have a preoccupation with leanness and muscularity, increases their desire to bulk up at all costs, even when they don't have the hormones to support it. It's troubling that so many children don't like their bodies. For all children a negative self-image informs their self-esteem, worthiness, and well-being, especially if they're growing up with a larger or smaller body.

We live in an appearance-focused, health-obsessed world, where societal standards about what it means to be "healthy" ring loud and clear. Often, larger and smaller kids don't fit into the social definition of "health" and are scrutinized and rated against these standards. If your child eats poorly, isn't an athlete, adores sweets, is hooked on social media, or isn't putting vegetables on their plate at mealtime, you, too, have a child who falls outside the norms of what it means to be "healthy." Unfortunately, society will blame *you*. Despite a real-world environment that encourages food at every turn, conveniences that sacrifice positive lifestyle habits, and other factors not under your control, *you* are held responsible for your child's size and habits.

An Impossible Choice: Restrict, Push, or Do Nothing

Ann was very concerned when she called me about her son Peter eight years ago. As we talked, it was clear Ann had a lot of skills and was tuned in to her child. She was a good cook who served family meals most nights. She and her husband were interested in nutrition for themselves but grappled with translating this into feeding their son.

Peter loved food, but Ann was concerned about his eating habits. He ate large amounts and was always the first one done, asking for more food. "I can tell he's gaining," she told me at one point. "He's eating more than his older brother, and I'm not sure what to do. It's hard to watch." She asked me whether she should teach him about nutrition, but worried this would backfire and send the wrong message. Peter wasn't athletically inclined or interested in sports, but she wondered if she should sign him up anyway. Ann was in that space many concerned parents find themselves, wanting to do something (because doing nothing meant things may get worse), but worried about doing it all wrong.

Like Ann, you may be faced with impossible choices every day. And it's not like you haven't tried to make things better. New recipes and sneaking veggies into smoothies and casseroles? Check. Healthier snacks? Yes. But you stop for a variety of reasons—it's expensive, time-consuming, your kid doesn't eat it and you're wasting food, or you're tired of the complaints. You know your child loves sweets and probably eats too many, so you've limited them, only to find your child overeating at parties, friends' houses, and school. When your child barely touches their food, you've reminded them to eat and threatened to remove their TV privileges, but it backfired with your kid dissolving into tears and ending the meal. So you go back to allowing more sweets than you're comfortable with or making your child what they want to eat in the hopes that it'll help. You know your child needs to exercise, but they complain and drag their feet, and you feel like a drill sergeant. And tame social media? That's a jungle for which you don't have a machete. Raising a kid with healthy habits? It all feels impossible!

> **#TruthBomb:**
> Fear that you may be missing an emerging health concern, or damaging your child's self-esteem, or creating more challenges for your child can leave many parents stuck in an uncomfortable limbo.

You've even tried subtle motivation, but it falls flat. You shudder at the thought of talking about size or the concerns about your child's health. You're not alone. Over a third of parents avoid talking with their children about their size due to fears of harming their self-esteem or causing an eating disorder. This number jumps to 65 percent when parents identify their child as larger. The last thing you want to do is make your kid feel bad or add problems.

The pressure to raise a healthy, trim, fit kid with healthy habits is overwhelming. You know the habits your child develops now are the habits they take into adulthood. The clock is ticking. So you promise to do something different. But you get up the next day and just don't have the energy. Life gets in the way. No matter what you do, you can't seem to get traction.

It's Harder Than Ever

You face many challenges as a parent: a world of abundant, accessible food; technology that encourages sitting around; a culture that emphasizes beauty, thinness, and fitness; "armchair experts" and professionals telling you what to do; children who are exposed to the pressures of society earlier and earlier. Additionally, social determinants of health, or the conditions of where you live, learn, work, and play, affect your child's health, quality of life, and risks, too. For instance, your economic stability affects what you can afford in the grocery store, and your neighborhood impacts whether your child can get outside and play, or get to sleep at night. While you're a primary influence on your child's physical health and emotional well-being, you're not the only factor. Ironically, many of the modern technologies and scientific advances we have today make raising healthy kids who feel good about themselves harder than ever.

"Every day I'm wracked with guilt that the way I'm dealing with my daughter's weight and her eating habits is wrong, doing more damage, and contributing to an adulthood where she may misunderstand the place food has in her life," wrote Kate in reply to my weekly newsletter. Questioning oneself and feeling guilty are par for the course.

If you have a smaller or larger child, you know that every parenting decision is that much harder. You'll ask yourself, *Should I encourage more food, or should I cut back? Should I sign them up for sports, or let them be? Should I try to change their size, or ignore it?* The questions about what to do never end. "We've got one child who is heavy and one who is thin," said Diane, mom to seven-year-old Blake and ten-year-old Ben. "It's impossible to plan dinners that will be good for both. We're telling Ben he's had enough, and telling Blake to eat more," she said. "I know I'm probably not handling this right, but I'm at a loss." Guilt and feelings of ineptness don't end, no matter the size of your child. The desire to raise your kid right, without causing harm, is one every parent feels. *So how do you raise a physically healthy child without causing emotional harm?* You need a clear path that addresses both goals.

But here's the thing: *Not even health professionals agree.* It turns out that health-care providers, educators, researchers, and anyone who cares about children and their health are asking this question, too.

The medical model, or what I call the Fix Size Model, considers size as a primary influence on health. On the opposite side, what I refer to as the Embrace Size Model believes that interventions to change body size cause harm. While both models embody the Hippocratic oath—*First, do no harm*—they embody this philosophy in different ways. Let's briefly look at each one.

The Fix Size Model: A Focus on Treatment

Fix Size seeks to change the bodies that are deemed to be too small or too large. The goal: support normal growth and improve body functioning. For kids who are larger, it means arresting or slowing down unhealthy weight gain by altering their diet or instituting more movement or other helpful lifestyle behaviors, so children can "grow into" their height. For those who are smaller, it may mean changing food or eating patterns to favor weight gain.

The Fix Size Model has plenty of research data to support its stance. For instance, there's an association between bodies with more adiposity (body fat) in childhood and the occurrence of type 2 diabetes, high blood pressure, fatty liver disease, high cholesterol, sleep apnea, and other respiratory problems later. The Fix Size Model attempts to address these negative health outcomes by improving lifestyle behaviors, such as incorporating more nutritious foods, limiting foods like desserts and high-fat foods, and encouraging more physical activity and better sleep habits.

> **#TruthBomb:**
> Despite the best of intentions, focusing on a child's size and physical health may harm their emotional well-being.

Fix Size asserts long-term health challenges can be reversed by changing body size (losing weight) and improving lifestyle behaviors. But, size reduction is not only hard to achieve, it's also very hard to sustain for the long haul, especially for children. The pursuit of long-term positive health outcomes may make children more vulnerable to collateral damage like poor self-esteem and metabolic damage from repeated efforts at weight loss. Children who are smaller in size and who aren't getting enough nutrition can experience effects on their mood, nutritional status, and physical health. Helping these kids change their size (gain weight) may come with its own set of consequences, namely, a disturbed relationship with food and eating.

The Embrace Size Model: A Focus on Emotional Well-Being

The Embrace Size Model does not see size as a problem. In fact, dieting or gaining weight to change one's size (or talking about size and poor health) feeds the roots of what this model believes is inherently problematic: a society that values thinness and health at the expense of psychological well-being. Embrace Size unites around fighting diet culture, a set of values that emphasize thinness, appearance, and size over health and well-being. Rallying against these, the Embrace Size Model believes interventions to change body size are more problematic than size itself, and are especially psychologically harmful to long-term health. Rather, the Fix Size Model focuses on behaviors that enhance health. Their goal: to preserve the well-being of the individual and avoid the emotional strain that stems from dieting and diet culture.

There is research that supports this perspective. For instance, older adults (sixty-five and older) who carry extra body fat do not have shorter life spans. Healthy lifestyle habits significantly decrease the risk of mortality (death), regardless of body size or body fat. And weight cycling, or the process of losing weight and then regaining it back, causes more harm to heart health than simply keeping body weight at a steady state. An emphasis on physical activity rather than weight loss may improve health and reduce mortality. And, when it comes to kids who are larger, a positive body image results in less weight gain five years later, according to research.

#TruthBomb: Positive lifestyle behaviors support the whole child, helping kids establish habits that encourage both physical health and emotional well-being.

The Embrace Size Model understands that pressures from diet culture cause anxiety, stress, and problematic eating. Social media, where diet culture is pervasive, has been implicated in body dissatisfaction, poor self-esteem, and eating disorders in children and teens. Embrace Size asks, *What's the benefit of addressing body size if it sacrifices a child's well-being?*

Both Fix Size and Embrace Size desire to help all children be well-nourished and physically and psychologically healthy. Although

Comparison of the Fix Size versus Embrace Size Models

Fix Size	Embrace Size
Prioritizes physical health	Prioritizes emotional well-being
Advocates for dietary and lifestyle changes to improve body function	Avoids restrictive diets, especially those promoting weight loss
Sees larger or smaller as a potential problem	Believes changing size, food, or eating may create health and emotional problems
Goal: change size and embrace health behaviors	*Goal*: embrace size and health behaviors

discord and disagreement exist over how this is accomplished, they *are* aligned in one area: positive lifestyle behaviors. Ultimately, the polarization of the two philosophies trickles down to parents and caregivers like you, making things more confusing. Confusion leads to indecision, which leads to inaction. Meanwhile, your child may miss out on the support they need the most. But even parents who *are* ready to act may still feel stuck. "I will do anything to help my daughter," said Kristen, a mom from Massachusetts. "But I don't know where to start. My doctor told me to get an app and have her start recording her food. Is that a good idea? I just don't know." Despite all the science, media coverage, and emerging treatments, the practical resources for parents, especially those who have children with larger bodies, are scant.

Online "How To" articles offer what to do (and not do) if your child is overeating, a picky eater, or gaining or losing weight. (I know, I've written some of these!) Many books center on food, offering recipes to help. Or they cover one aspect of eating, like intuition, adventurousness, overeating, or picky eating. Apps that track eating aren't necessarily the answer, either, as they may draw too much focus to food. None of these available resources cover *everything* you need to know and do to start helping your child grow up healthy, inside and out.

The Impossible Is Possible

Many of the families I've seen over the years have tried everything . . . and nothing had worked. With desperation rooted in confusion, frustration, societal pressures, and the nagging feeling that health problems would be part of their child's future, they looked for answers and a better way. My first call with Ann was the beginning of a relationship that progressively addressed proven lifestyle behaviors, one by one. First, we directed our attention to their family culture, as she wanted to make sure Peter felt accepted, respected, and secure within their family. We looked at the language used and perspectives about food, bodies, and eating; they reflected on their food history and how it showed up in their parenting; and we improved how the family interacted around mealtimes. We then turned to food, revamping the food balance, planning nutritious meals and snacks, and building more structure around sweets and treats. Peter was a fast eater, so Ann implemented strategies to slow him down and teach him mindfulness and pace with eating. One by one, we tackled all the lifestyle behaviors. Ann encouraged Peter to explore different sports and activities offered by his school, adopting an attitude of adventure, fun, and learning. Peter found he had many interests, especially tennis and strength training. He was a great sleeper and loved to read, so screen time wasn't a challenge, but Ann understood the role they played in Peter's overall health and was committed to tending to them as he grew. My work with Peter highlights a whole-child approach, addressing lifestyle behaviors: Family culture. Sleep. Movement. Feeding. Eating. Food. Screens. Self-care. I've always used these, which I call the 8 Pillars of Wellness, oftentimes with different priorities, to address the needs of the child and family.

Today, Peter is a teenager. He enjoys working out, can cook, and by all accounts lives a healthier lifestyle than most of his peers. He's grown into his body and he's physically healthy, but more important, he's confident, secure, and feels good about himself. In my thirty-plus years as a pediatric dietitian, this has always been my goal: to empower parents to create an environment that nourishes and nurtures their children, without creating an emotional toll, and to help children grow up physically healthy, functioning well, and feeling good about themselves at every size.

In my career, I've helped families whose children had larger and smaller bodies, eating disorders, and health conditions. Most of these families felt lost when they came to me, but with the right tools and knowledge, they felt empowered. I've learned and gained insight from my pediatric training and work, from counseling real families, and as a mom. I've learned from the research and the experts who've joined me on my podcast, and from the medical model and the Health at Every Size® approach, both of which I use in my practice. But the polarization between these models only muddies the water, confusing parents like you who want to do right by their child. I know there's a better way—a meeting of the minds—and that's how I came to an approach that considers the *whole child*.

Addressing the Whole Child

t's time for a fresh approach that addresses both the physical health and emotional well-being of the *whole child*. A path for cultivating healthful behaviors in *every* child. One that takes the science and principles of health behaviors and transforms them into a system that helps you cultivate a variety of healthful habits, regardless of your child's size.

Kids Thrive at Every Size is an operating manual—a road map—for navigating the ins and outs of raising children who are larger, smaller, or in-between. Drawn from science and experts in medicine, psychology, exercise, sleep, media, and nutrition, this book not only helps you establish healthful habits, but it delivers a heightened awareness of the social issues, health concerns, and psychological impact of growing up in today's culture, especially when larger or smaller. Just like assembling a piece of furniture, you need all the bits and pieces and a good

> **#TruthBomb:** All children, no matter their size, need to develop and participate in a variety of healthful behaviors and attitudes. These become the roots of positive lifestyle habits, influencing future health and well-being.

instruction manual. If you don't have all of these, putting together your new desk will feel impossible (and it will be). Similarly, *Kids Thrive at Every Size* lays out a holistic approach with the most important lifestyle behaviors you need to raise a healthy child, inside and out. It all begins with what I call the Whole-Child Healthy model.

The Whole-Child Healthy Model

The Whole-Child Healthy model places equal emphasis on your child's physical health *and* emotional well-being. It rests on a belief that it's possible to nourish and nurture children simultaneously as they grow and develop, resulting in kids who grow up physically *and* emotionally well. Using this "nourish and nurture" approach solves the conundrums of achieving physical health while avoiding emotional harm and cultivating emotional well-being without sacrificing physical health. Whole-Child Healthy is a model for all children, of *every* size.

Whole-Child Healthy is a prevention approach, helping you set up specific health habits to support your child from an early age as they grow. It can also be the guide if you need to reset health behaviors in your home. Whole-Child Healthy relies on the latest research while keeping things practical and user-friendly. It has several core tenets:

- ♥ *Every* body is a growing, good body, no matter its shape or size.
- ♥ All children need to build health-enhancing lifestyle habits, no matter their size.
- ♥ Enjoyment is fundamental to health and well-being.
- ♥ Children learn, grow, and change, and their parents need to be aware of the changes, support them, and adapt.
- ♥ Parents are role models and the gatekeepers of myriad influences on their children and should be fully empowered to lead their children to health and well-being.
- ♥ Children are respected, engaged, and protected on all levels.

The Whole-Child Healthy model knows that all children benefit from healthy habits and behaviors, but *how* we instill these, and educate, and help children implement them, makes all the difference. With a sensitivity to child development, temperament, and readiness, the Whole-Child Healthy model takes a wide lens, recognizing there's more to raising healthy, secure children than the mainstream advice of a healthy meal or daily movement. It's about nourishing the whole child with all foods, positive eating experiences, movement, and sleep while nurturing the child's relationship with food, eating, and self through the family culture, feeding, and the active cultivation of self-love. And this is where the 8 Pillars of Wellness are key.

The 8 Pillars of Wellness

The backbone of the Whole-Child Healthy model is the key health behaviors that promote and protect your child's health and well-being. I call these the 8 Pillars of Wellness. They focus on the most important influences on your child's developing health and well-being. They are:

- ♥ Family Culture
- ♥ Sleep
- ♥ Movement
- ♥ Feeding
- ♥ Eating
- ♥ Food
- ♥ Screens
- ♥ Self-Love

Like the foundation of a building, each Pillar needs to be strong and deeply rooted to stand the test of time. From cultivating a positive family culture to understanding the power of sleep, each of these Pillars provides a guide to formulating positive health behaviors from an early age. The Whole-Child Healthy model and the 8 Pillars of Wellness will make you a whole lot wiser—in fact, Size Wise—making the path to raising a healthy and happy child crystal clear.

Whole-Child Healthy Understands	Whole-Child Healthy Cultivates
• Physical and emotional development need equal emphasis. • Key health behaviors are foundational to health and well-being. • Psychological vulnerabilities exist for all children, but especially for the larger and smaller child. • Parents are primary facilitators of children's health behaviors. • There's a healthy person in *every* child. • Small behavioral changes over time lead to dramatic improvements in health and well-being. • *Every* body is a good body.	• A child with a strong body and sense of self. • Health habits that can last a lifetime. • Confident parents who have a clear understanding and path for raising a healthy child, inside and out. • A holistic, inclusive, whole-child approach to health. • Connected families and secure children.

The Size Wise Parent Understands	The Size Wise Parent Cultivates
• Health includes physical functioning and emotional well-being. • Behaviors form habits and habits inform future health. • Kids come in all shapes and sizes. • Genetics create the blueprint; environment influences health outcomes. • There's more to raising a healthy kid than good food and exercise. • Children's emotional well-being needs protection, especially when bodies are larger or smaller. • Enjoyment is foundational to wellness. • Diet culture is a danger to emotional well-being.	• A structured, positive, nurturing home environment. • Opportunities for a variety of healthful lifestyle behaviors. • A shame-free, inclusive home. • A model of lifestyle behaviors that promote overall health and well-being.

Why You Need This Book

Research tells us about physical health and mental well-being, but nobody has put together a resource for raising healthy kids who feel good about themselves no matter their size. Nor has anybody delivered a solution that strikes when the iron is hot—during the preschool to preteen years, when establishing habits and self-esteem is easiest. *Kids Thrive at Every Size* lets you break away from tired messages like "eat less, move more," and focus on the behaviors that truly help your child establish good habits without psychological consequences.

Kids Thrive at Every Size details *how* to set up health behaviors with added guidance if your child is smaller or larger. The focus is on your child and your family system, encouraging you to implement small changes that stack up to big results. You will encounter information that's "good to know," nerdy science to offer you a deeper understanding, and other advice that you'll find eye-opening and fundamentally critical to helping your child. I know that every child and family is different, and my goal is to give you information and options. Take what you need. And know that you've got a resource as your child grows.

From preschool to preteen, *Kids Thrive at Every Size* gives you an implementable plan, helps you overcome common obstacles, and highlights practical strategies for healthful lifestyle behaviors. Most important, *Kids Thrive at Every Size* answers the most significant question you have: *How do I help my child grow up healthy without harming them along the way?*

How to Use This Book

I've divided *Kids Thrive at Every Size* into two parts. In Part 1, you'll learn the basics about physical health and emotional well-being. I'll cover the genetics of size and growth; the tools that evaluate your child's health; and conditions that may influence your child's organ function, metabolism, and health outcomes. Additionally, you'll learn about how your child's mind and social-emotional health develop, and how these influence their self-esteem, worthiness, and body satisfaction. These are the building blocks of the Whole-Child Healthy model. Health and well-being are connected, both influencing the other as your child grows and develops, and they provide the basis for entering Part 2 of this book.

In Part 2, you'll be introduced to the 8 Pillars of Wellness: family culture, sleep, movement, feeding, eating, food, screens, and self-love. These are the key habits and attitudes you'll need to raise a healthy, happy child, especially if they have a larger or smaller body. Within each Pillar of Wellness, I break down the science about each health behavior, cover the obstacles that prohibit the development of each habit, and provide practical advice on how to cultivate positive behaviors, whether you're just starting out or are well on your way. Throughout this section, I tease out specific information for children with smaller and larger bodies. My goal is to help you define age-appropriate, developmentally sensitive, small, repeatable changes. Over time, these become your child's habits.

At the end of each chapter, you'll have a chance to evaluate how you're doing in each Pillar with a screening tool called *The Whole-Child Checkup*. Based on a rating scale of *Learner*, *Striver*, or *Thriver*, you'll get clarity on how you're doing and a focus area to work on (and by the end of the book, you may have several!). For example, if you identify as a *Learner*, that Pillar will be an area where you'll want to make changes. If you're a *Striver*, you're on the right track. You'll be asked to level up those health behaviors with specific suggestions. If you're a *Thriver*, you're all set. No need to work on this; just keep doing what you're doing. But you'll be encouraged to keep your eye on things as your child grows. As a result of knowing how you're doing in each Pillar, you'll understand where you need to focus your attention. No more *"I don't know where to begin!"*

I've put the Pillars in the order in which I believe they'll be most impactful, but you can tackle any Pillar in the order that benefits you most. If you are struggling in one particular Pillar, feel free to go there first. And, of course, if you find my suggestions aren't working for your child, you don't have to implement them. The spirit of this book is to give you options, not instill blame or harm your child. The final chapter takes the self-assessments from each Pillar and brings them together as a master blueprint for moving forward. This will help you see your strengths and priority areas of improvement. You'll also get a suggested method for tackling other health behaviors I haven't covered in the book. I'll answer a few Frequently Asked Questions (FAQs) and offer you some parting words of wisdom. All the references are in the back, and supportive resources can be found in the Appendix. Building lifestyle habits is a long game! Keep this book handy so you can refer back for guidance, get inspired to tackle something new, or unravel unhelpful habits.

My aim is to show you how to set up a healthy home environment, one Pillar at a time, imprinting a way of life that encourages physical health and emotional well-being, no matter your child's size. I hope you feel like Ann did—empowered—and learn that raising healthy and happy children of *every* size is possible and attainable. Let me show you how!

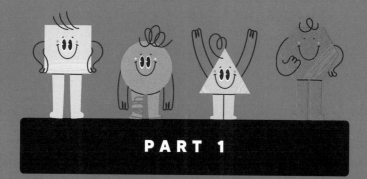

PART 1

Health is a state of complete physical, mental, and social well-being and not merely the absence of disease or infirmity.

—WORLD HEALTH ORGANIZATION, 1948

The Building Blocks of Health

Seventh grade. One of the worst years of my childhood. By the time I was twelve, I was long-limbed and knobby-kneed, with nary a sign of puberty. I had a serious overbite and braces. I wore headgear 24/7, little rubber bands that ran tracks through my mouth, and glasses. I was smaller in size and a late bloomer. I was called "freckle face," "four eyes," "bucky," and some other slurs I've worked hard to forget. Name-calling was relatively tame in the seventies compared to today, but it still hurt. I *felt* like the ugliest girl in the world.

As a mom, I've navigated the decade between preschool and the end of middle school with my own four children. I recall the intensity of teaching and reinforcing manners at the table, setting rules and routines, and the relentless negotiations around bedtimes, Game Boys, and sleepovers. I also remember my own worries about whether my kids were healthy and happy; calling on my inner "Mama Bear" when my kids were bullied or left out (and they all were at some point or another); and supporting them through disappointments, failures, and rejection. The truth is, all kids change physically, emotionally, and cognitively during this time, and these changes threaten their physical health and emotional well-being. And it doesn't help that they're increasingly vulnerable to others' opinions and impressions.

Today, my kids are young adults, and I've been a pediatric dietitian for over thirty years. What I've witnessed during this time is both encouraging and discouraging. I'm impressed with the education parents have about nutrition today, but I'm astounded that we've slowly but surely let our children's emotional well-being take a backseat to an idealized notion of health. This has cost us and our kids.

What is real health? Many believe health is rooted in appearance (size) and eating habits. But it's not. For true health, your child needs both a functioning body and a sense of happiness with themself and their world. In equal parts.

My greatest gift to my clients has been the ability to offer them support, understanding of their child, and comprehensive knowledge about what it means to pursue true health in childhood. This chapter aims to do the same. To truly help your child, you need to have knowledge of these physical changes and stages of development so you can stay one step ahead. Of course, this isn't easy! One, your child is constantly changing. By the time you've got one stage figured out, your child changes and you have to adapt. Two, life marches on. At the end of the day, no matter how worried you may be about your child's health, size, or emotional well-being, you still need to make dinner, get your kid to bed, and off to school the next day.

In other words, life happens alongside these changes and challenges. If food, daily habits, and your child's size are worrisome, you may not have the luxury of putting life on hold to address them. But with greater insight into these building blocks, you can anticipate and change with your child, and navigate concerns if and when they do come up.

Kids come in all shapes and sizes. Some kids are tall and lean, others are stout and sturdy. Some carry more muscle, and others have more fat. They also have an innate temperament, and at any point in time, they're in a state of cognitive, social, and emotional development that governs much of their thinking, actions, and motivations. Because the body and brain change so much in this decade, we'll consider the key building blocks that promote physical health and emotional well-being for the *whole child*.

Physical Health: Genetics, Growth, and Puberty

"My daughter, who is now six, started gaining weight between ages two and three, in her belly, which seemed very odd at the time," said Hanalee, a mom and nurse from Utah. "It was obvious, but I just chalked it up to a growth spurt on its way." Over time, Hanalee's daughter continued to grow larger. "It's been a mystery to me. I don't carry extra body fat and her two siblings don't either. Overall, I'm just perplexed."

Why is it that some children are chubby from the day they are born? They carry more body fat than their siblings, yet live in the same home and eat the same food. Why are some kids ahead of the pack in their development? And why are others late bloomers? I wish I could state that it has everything to do with what and how much your child eats, but that's not necessarily the case. Some kids are naturally lean, some have a larger frame, and some are born naturally carrying more body fat. Why is that? The answer is *genetics*.

Your child's body blueprint was determined before you ever met. The mixing of the X and Y chromosomes created a DNA expression that determined your child's hair, eye, and skin color. It also determined your child's basic shape and size—even the amount of body fat and muscle they tend to carry—and where it's placed on their body. Just like your child's height, size is an inherited trait.

Across gender and age, there is a 40-50 percent likelihood of inheriting a genetic trait for body fat and size. Some studies indicate it's even

> **#TruthBomb:** Height is 80 percent heritable. If you took a large group of people and compared their height, most (80 percent) of the difference between them would be attributable to their genes. The rest of what makes them tall (or not) is caused by other factors, like nutrition.

higher, up to 85 percent in certain cases. Interestingly, identical twins raised apart have a 70 percent heritability rate for size, regardless of the environment in which they grow up. But genes aren't your child's destiny. Body size is also influenced by the lifestyle your child leads, such as their eating habits, physical activity, and sleep patterns. And that's what this book is all about—cultivating the conditions and behaviors that help your child, no matter their size and genetic tendency, grow up healthy, inside and out. The following chart offers a rough guide of the varying sizes in childhood.

The Size Spectrum

	Smaller	Midsize	Larger
Height	Short or average	Average	Tall or average
Weight	Lower or average body fat and/or muscle	Average body fat and/or muscle	More body fat and/or muscle
Frame	Petite, small-boned	Average	Broad, big-boned

Growth and Puberty

Growth is the process whereby the body increases in physical size up to adulthood. Arms and legs lengthen, torsos widen and stretch, and the head grows larger. Of course, the internal organs develop, too. The two fastest periods of growth in childhood are infancy and adolescence. At these times, the pace of growth accelerates. During toddlerhood and the elementary school years, growth is slow and steady. When puberty rolls around, a second uptick in growth occurs. Known as the adolescent growth spurt, this is when hormones, including growth hormone, testosterone, estrogen and progesterone, and others, promote a rapid pace of growth, resulting in increased height and weight gain.

Puberty typically begins between ages eight and thirteen in girls, and nine and fourteen in boys. Many parents start to get concerned as they watch this stage unfold because there's quite a bit of body weight and height gain. Mary approached me about her daughter Rebecca.

She was nine years old and gaining weight around her middle. "Her belly's getting bigger," said Mary. "She's active and seems to eat well, and thankfully she's not worried about it, but I'm a little concerned." I reassured Mary that gaining body fat in the midsection is completely normal at this stage. Girls gain weight, particularly in the tummy area, before they start their period. As they get taller, their body weight

EARLY AND LATE BLOOMERS

Puberty has been occurring earlier in children over the last two decades, by about twelve to eighteen months. Evidence suggests girls with more body fat may experience early puberty and begin their period sooner, but the reasons why aren't clear. Early puberty might also be explained by endocrine-disrupting chemicals, such as those found in pesticides and food. Even genetic influences, like whether or not you were an early or late bloomer, may affect the timing of your child's puberty.

Precocious puberty is defined as puberty onset *before age eight* in girls and *before age nine* in boys. It's more common in girls and includes breast buds development, increased height growth and skeletal maturity, enlargement of the ovaries and uterus, and increased hormone levels. If your child has hair growth or body odor at a young age, they may have partial puberty or what is called premature pubarche. It's a form of incomplete puberty, mostly demonstrated by early pubic hair. More than 4 percent of young girls experience this and over half of them carry higher amounts of body fat. While each child's "blooming time" will be unique, there is also the late bloomer to consider. In girls, delayed puberty is defined as a lack of breast bud development by age thirteen, and no period by age sixteen. For boys, delayed puberty is suspected when there are no signs of testicular maturation, voice deepening, and pubic hair before age fourteen. If you're concerned about your child's pubertal progression, talk with your pediatrician.

redistributes, and the addition of fat tissue—to the rear, hips, breasts, backs of arms, and thighs—occurs. If you notice your daughter is blossoming in size, remember that it's part of the natural progression to womanhood.

It's also typical for boys to appear thicker during the preteen years. As testosterone levels rise, their muscles begin to grow, becoming defined and larger. For many preteen boys, the pudginess you see will decrease and shift to other areas of the body, and they will stretch into their adult height. Of course, some children won't appear fleshy during this time at all. They'll remain slim, and you may wonder when puberty will happen. There are lots of variabilities! Understanding this means you won't overreact to the expected changes of puberty.

Growth Charts, Curves, and Body Mass Index (BMI)

Since your child's arrival, you've been heading to the pediatrician's office for an annual checkup. During these visits, your doctor makes note of your child's growth by measuring weight and height and plotting them on standardized growth charts for your child's age and gender. These charts were designed to compare your child to a reference population. The value of these is not in comparing your child to every other kid in the world, but in using the chart as a gauge for measuring your child *against their own growth progress* over time. In general, kids track predictably along one channel or percentile range year over year after toddlerhood. When your child wavers from their usual growth pattern, it's time to look deeper.

Fluctuations—up or down—may happen, and they may or may not be problematic. For example, a child may jump from one channel to a higher one on their weight curve, from the 40th percentile to the 85th percentile, or they may fall off their height curve, tailing off from the 25th percentile to the 10th percentile. Changes in growth like these can alert you or your health-care provider to look more closely at habits and lifestyle behaviors. But don't panic. Many kids fluctuate in their growth, especially during puberty. You can locate growth charts for your child at www.cdc.gov/growthcharts.

You've probably heard about the body mass index, or BMI. It's yet another tool health-care providers use to measure your child's growth.

Specifically, BMI measures whether your child's body mass (weight) is at a reasonable level for how tall (height) they are. BMI values are categorized as "underweight," "healthy weight," "overweight," and "obese." Initially developed for scientific studies of populations, not individuals, it's considered a proxy for body fat levels, but it has several shortcomings. One, it fails to differentiate the body composition of fat, muscle, or bone. As such, BMI can misclassify a child who is naturally more muscular or built in a larger frame as "overweight." Two, BMI may suggest a child is at a "healthy weight" when, in fact, their body composition favors more fat mass than lean tissue.

#WiseAdvice: *Normal growth* is a term that should be interpreted with caution. Every child's rate of growth is individualized based on genetics, nutrition, and other environmental factors. Even though we have "norms," a child's normal growth pattern is unique to them. Don't compare your child to anyone else.

There are more issues with BMI, especially as a tool to measure physical health. I encourage you to take it with a grain of salt. Much like the growth chart, the BMI and BMI growth curves may be useful tools for tracking your child's growth and how they're developing over time. But they aren't the Holy Grail. By far the biggest issue with BMI is its inability to represent the bigger picture—your child's *functional* health. Plus, interpretations of BMI may increase the risk of stigma and harm, especially for children with smaller and larger bodies. It may

WATCHING YOUR CHILD'S HEIGHT

Short stature (a height for age that is less than the 3rd percentile) or a noticeable slowing of growth on the height curve may or may not be a problem. There are many reasons for being shorter in stature, including genetic factors, lack of nutrition, growth hormone deficiency, or a delay in pubertal development. If you're concerned, talk with your pediatrician, who may consult with an endocrinologist.

point health-care providers and parents down the path of "fixing" size, which can lead to other problems with body image, self-esteem, and worthiness.

Your child's growth charts should be interpreted carefully by a professional and discussed with you, *not your child*. In fact, some parents keep a sticky note in their child's medical record explicitly requesting all conversations about weight, BMI, and health *do not occur in front of their child*. But for better or worse, the growth charts can help you understand how your child's individual growth is evolving over time. Remember, these are just *tools*. They aren't the be-all and end-all indicator of your child's health. When they are use to problematize a child's size, they can cause harm. They are not representations of who your child is or how healthy (or not) they are. Remember, your child's growth assessment is not a grade, it's simply a small piece of their bigger health picture.

Takeaways:

- Your child's growth and timing of puberty are dependent on a number of factors, including their genetic makeup and environment. It's expected to see more weight gain and growth during puberty.

- Growth charts allow you to track your child's individual growth over time.

- The growth and BMI-for-age charts are singular tools for tracking your child's physical growth. There are other determinants of your child's health and body functioning.

Well-Being: Cognitive, Social, and Emotional Development

Your child's emotional well-being is the counterpart to their physical health—something we do not emphasize enough, in my opinion. This is what makes this book unique—it is a look at your child's overall health through the lens of both physical health and emotional well-being.

Not only do kids' bodies evolve and change as they grow up, their brains do, too. How your child thinks and matures provides insight into many things, including how to shape their lifestyle behaviors. As they grow and change, you can anticipate their choices, behaviors, and motivations. If you can't, you'll feel like you're losing control and influence over them, or be confused and frustrated by their actions. The key to staying one step ahead of your child is understanding their social, emotional, and cognitive changes over time.

How Your Child Thinks (Cognitive Development)

Cognitive development is all about the brain and how it thinks. Children's brains undergo tremendous development between the ages of two and seven years. During this critical period, neurons in the brain connect to each other, creating an "information highway," which allows kids to learn quickly—twice as fast as at any other time of life. In fact, young children have twice as many neural connections as adults do. Yes, "kids are like sponges." They soak up information through a back-and-forth engagement with their environment, which cements these neural connections and circuitry. As such, this is the time to expose young children to a wide variety of activities, help them develop a love of learning, and teach them to identify and describe their emotions.

During the school-age years (ages 6–12), the brain is nearly (90–95 percent) the size of the adult brain. While most neural connections are formed in the early years, they're still being built at this time. However, around the preteen years and into adolescence, pruning begins, a process wherein neurons are eliminated and refined, like cutting back a plant to encourage fuller growth. Pruning enhances the neural pathways and prioritizes the circuits for learning, language, and other skills, like remembering how to do a math problem or knowing the steps to make pancakes. In adolescence, pruning kicks into high gear, and the brain circuits are essentially reorganized. (This is why teens can be so unpredictable, impulsive, and disorganized!)

"Getting buy-in and engagement from my tween is my biggest struggle," said Amelia, mom to a ten-year-old daughter. "I'm looking for a balance between instilling a belief that health matters, being positive and constructive, versus scaring, scolding, demeaning, shaming, guilting, and fighting about being healthy." How your child thinks—and how this evolves—is called cognitive development. As children grow, their intelligence grows, as does their mental model of the world around them. There are four stages of cognitive development based on the work of psychologist Jean Piaget: sensorimotor (birth to two years), preoperational (two to seven years), concrete operational (seven to eleven years), and formal operational (twelve years and up). These four stages occur sequentially in each child, but not necessarily at the same rate. As your child moves through these stages, how they think matures, but their social and cultural influences and environment also play a role.

You may wonder why your child's cognitive development matters. Mostly, it tells you about their readiness to learn, understand, and adopt desirable behaviors. Take Sam, who brought his eight-year-old son Brendon to see me years ago. Sam was frustrated by his son's "unhealthy" eating and wanted me to motivate him to eat better. His lectures weren't working. He thought if Brendon understood nutrition, then naturally, he would be inspired to make changes. But Brendon's ability to understand nutrition was limited, as it is for most kids his age. Although he understood the food groups, he didn't fully grasp the connection between food and later health. Nor was he willing to change his eating habits based on this information. Instead, Brendon needed more opportunities to interact with food, such as making his own snack, or learning how to make a salad or prep vegetables. He needed to see and live in a nutritious food environment, interact with it, and absorb the food lessons that came naturally. This was more likely to engage, motivate, and stick with him.

Cognitive Developmental Stages

Stage	Characteristics	Examples
Preoperational **(2 to 7 years)**	Egocentrism; illogical thinking; symbolism and role playing; magical thinking; parallel play	Cannot take the viewpoint of others, though some researchers believe children as young as 4 years show empathy. Taking on the role of "mommy" in pretend play. Using a broomstick to represent a horse. Early play is side-by-side and becomes interactive as the child ages.
Concrete Operational **(7 to 11 years)**	Logical thinking; concrete thinking; inductive reasoning; reversibility; conservation; less egocentrism	Can take a specific situation and generalize it. Thinks in extremes: good food and bad food or bad guy and good guy. Can determine a bag of candy shared among two people is still one bag of candy. Can see all aspects of a problem rather than just focus on one aspect.
Formal Operational **(12 years and up)**	Abstract thinking and reasoning about hypothetical problems; theoretical thinking; systematic planning	Has creative ideas and logical solutions for problems. Can think about bigger topics. Can plan ahead and predict outcomes and consequences.

EXECUTIVE FUNCTIONING SKILLS AND BEHAVIOR

W hy do kids grab another child's toy without asking? Or overindulge in cake and candy at a birthday party? How do they learn to control their behavior? They need to rely on their executive functioning skills or the "management system" in their brain. Executive function is a set of cognitive skills that develop over time as your child grows, much like cognition and intelligence. Examples of executive functioning skills include paying attention in the classroom, starting a task and finishing it, organizing and planning a future event, regulating emotions, and keeping track of and controlling activities.

The three main areas of executive functioning are working memory, flexible thinking, and self-control. *Working memory* allows your child to remember and use information over short periods of time. *Flexible thinking* means your child can shift their thinking or attention depending on different demands or rules. *Self-control* is the ability to change priorities and resist impulsive actions or responses. Flexible thinking and self-control, especially, are important areas to consider as you help your child build healthy behaviors.

Children may have high or low self-control. High self-control means a child can control their behavior in a variety of settings. They're more likely to follow the rules and wait for a reward, for example. Children with low self-control may demonstrate impulsive behaviors, like overeating when preferred foods are available or interrupting the teacher in the classroom. Children growing up in poverty or from other very high-risk backgrounds may lag in their development of executive functioning skills. Additionally, up to 40–50 percent of children with attention-deficit/hyperactivity disorder (ADHD) may have lower self-control. As you dive deeper into this book, keep your child's executive functioning skills in mind. If your child seems "out of control," they may need more time to develop these skills or more support in this area.

How Your Child Relates and Feels (Social-Emotional Development)

Your child's social-emotional development—their understanding and expression of emotions and how they interact with other people—unfolds over a series of stages throughout their childhood. At each stage of social-emotional development, children face a conflict that offers a turning point in their development. If they master the psychological strength of the stage, they proceed to the next stage of development. If they fail or poorly achieve the milestone, they may get stuck, hindering their next stage and impacting their emerging sense of self.

Preschoolers are meant to learn initiative—the sense of control over their environment and the ability to plan, start a task, or face a challenge. As a young preschooler, one of my daughters used to say, "I have a oog idea!" (a good idea). Anytime she wanted to be part of the conversation or insert her opinions, she would use this phrase. She was showing initiative. Responding with "Yes, I like that idea!" or "What if we did it this way?" reinforced her sense of purpose and the psychological strength of this stage, and supported her progression to the next stage. If I had ignored her or didn't validate her contribution to the conversation, she might have learned guilt and shame. These feelings could instill a fear of trying new things or sharing new ideas, diminishing her agency. Of course, developing a sense of purpose in the preschool years is the goal, and it happens with many interactions over time, not just one situation. As kids enter school, the goalpost moves. They need to learn industriousness to build confidence in themselves. To do so, they need ample and varied opportunities to build skills, from making cookies and washing dishes to cooperating on a team and standing up for themselves. Moving through each psychological stage successfully leads to the strengthening of one's sense of self while the opposite may lead to a sense of inadequacy or poor self-esteem.

The stages of social-emotional development occur predictably, much like the stages of cognitive development. For the purpose of this book, we'll focus on the following: initiative, industry, and the beginnings of identity.

Initiative: This is the stage most three- to five-year-olds are in. Their goal is to develop purpose. They do this by pushing for autonomy, testing limits, and learning flexible self-control. The standoff at the dinner table and on the potty has a purpose! This is a good time to set limits and offer choices (and let your child make the choice) to support their autonomy and initiative.

Industry: From ages six to eleven, the goal is to build confidence and a sense of industry. Providing rules and directions, assigning responsibilities, and teaching social skills, like apologizing or speaking up, helps children develop self-confidence. I assure you, assigning chores and expecting help from your child is good parenting and an advantage for their development. Friends take on significant importance during this

WHY EARLY ATTACHMENT IS SO IMPORTANT

Social-emotional development begins and flows from secure attachment, which develops during infancy when parents and babies establish a bond. Attachment is based on a caregiver's responsiveness to their child's needs, whereby the caretaker anticipates and responds to the infant's cues. Over time, if needs have been met, the infant develops trust and a secure attachment to the caregiver. Without secure attachment, the next stages of social-emotional development may be disrupted. More important, secure attachment allows children to seek their caregiver in times of stress and lays the foundation of a child's sense of security, self-esteem, self-regulation, and self-control. "We are born with strong emotions and no ability to know what to do with them," says Dr. Serena Messina, a psychologist and researcher who conducted studies at the University of Texas at Austin. "But within interactions with a sensitive caregiver, children learn to name their emotions. They learn what to do when they have feelings." A secure attachment is the first stage of psychological development and is the backbone of parent-child trust, and a sense of self.

time of life, and your child will make more decisions on their own and desire independence. Praise, affection, and setting up a balance between rules and independence promote self-confidence and self-assurance.

Identity: The preteen years (and into the older teen years) is a time of identity development. The preteen child may not be as self-aware as we would hope, but they are moving forward in building their identity. They're vulnerable to opinions and other influences, and may internalize these to answer the big question of "Who am I?" If you're hoping your child will be motivated to improve their health, this stage may be frustrating. Be patient. Their motivation relies on self-identity, which fully blooms later in adolescence. In the meantime, supportive adult relationships are key, particularly now, as children may experience bullying and friendship woes.

How Your Child Reacts (Temperament)

Temperament is something your child is born with—it's hardwired and characterizes your child's approach and interaction with the world. Temperament is often described as your child's "style" or "personality." It informs how your child might react to situations and others, and what their disposition might be like. Researchers generally categorize children into three main temperament categories. These categories are broad, so your child may not fit exactly into one of these, but they can help you better identify your child's strengths and needs. They are:

Easy or flexible: Your child is friendly, easygoing, complies with routines, adapts to change, and has a calm disposition.

Active or feisty: Your child is fussy, doesn't follow routines easily, is irregular with eating and sleeping, is apprehensive about changes or newness (including people), reacts intensely, and is easily upset.

Slow to warm up or cautious: Your child is shy, especially with new people or situations, is less engaged or active, may withdraw or have negative reactions, but becomes more comfortable with repeated exposure.

Imagine how temperament plays out with food and eating, a desire to be active (or not), and the willingness to follow routines at home and in school. For instance, the child who is cautious may need several exposures to a new food to warm up and try it, while the easygoing child may dive in without protest. Or the feisty child may be resistant to routines like bedtime or limits on media use, while the slow-to-warm-up child just needs to repeatedly engage in the routine to make it a mainstay. If you understand your child's temperament, you can be sensitive to their needs, especially when setting up desirable behaviors.

The Development of Self-Esteem

Your child's social-emotional development and temperament feed their self-esteem. Good self-esteem generally means your child regards themself as worthy, is happy, and is willing to take initiative. Positive self-esteem is a basic feature of mental health and a protective factor of physical health and social behavior. Poor self-esteem, on the other hand, is tied to mental health concerns and social problems, such as anxiety, depression, eating disorders, violence, substance abuse, and high-risk behaviors.

Children need approval, support, and a sense of competence to develop self-esteem. Attachment, unconditional love, and support from caregivers are critical. When children learn new skills, have new experiences, interact with their environment, and receive acknowledgment and validation, they have a greater likelihood of developing strong self-esteem. If they see themselves as competent, this boosts it. But the opposite—criticism, low acceptance, parental depression, maltreatment, and family discord and disruption—can cause poor self-esteem.

Helping a child build self-esteem involves giving them ample opportunity to build skills, garner validation, and a warm environment in which to learn. Here's a recipe for how to do that:

Skill-building: Let your child cook, garden, or complete household tasks. These offer a natural way to enhance skills, reinforce competency, and build self-esteem. Co-planning meals, working out a family media plan, and co-developing the family routines are good examples. You don't have to orchestrate elaborate experiences. Use your everyday environment to teach skills of daily living.

Ways to Promote Your Child's Self-Esteem

Action	Examples
Speak to and listen to your child with respect.	"Would you do [xyz]?" "Thank you for being [xyz]." "Can I get your input on [xyz]?"
Give attention and affection freely.	Look your child in the eyes during conversations. Hugs, kisses, and appropriate physical contact are ways to connect.
Help your child learn skills.	Teach your child life skills, such as how to dress and undress themself, wash the dishes, set the table, take out the trash, do their own laundry, groom the dog, ride a bike, etc.
Avoid harsh criticism and negative talk about others and yourself.	Don't say "I/You forget everything!" when you/your child make(s) a mistake or forget(s) something.
Focus on inner qualities and strengths.	Honor loyalty, persistence, attention to detail, being a confidant and friend, thoughtfulness, truthfulness, intelligence, etc.
Praise your child's effort, progress, and attitude (remember, overpraise rings hollow).	"I noticed how much time and effort you put into building that fort!" "You always get up with a happy attitude—you really brighten my day." "I know how frustrating this must feel, but I'm proud of you for seeing this through."

Validation: Praise helps cultivate self-esteem, but this may be overdone when parents give elaborate or empty praise. Psychologists agree that praise alone is not the path to self-esteem. In fact, empty praise, or praise that is ingenuine, like telling your child they're the next Picasso (when they're an average artist), or praise that focuses on the person—instead of the process—may cause more shame, especially if failure is involved. It's the difference between "You're a great artist!" (personal praise) and "You did a great job at drawing so much detail on that tree!" (process praise).

Warmth: Homes with warm and responsive parents, a "learning" environment, and a safe, organized physical environment are key elements to developing positive self-esteem in childhood—even well into adulthood. Unresponsive or inattentive parents and a chaotic home undermine a child's self-esteem. Some children learn that in order to be worthy or loved, they need to be perfect.

Now that you've learned about how your child develops during this decade of life and all the other things that feed into how they operate in the world, you may feel like a mini-psychologist! But understanding this part of your child's development allows you to be more sensitive when establishing healthful behaviors.

Takeaways:

- Your child's development influences their thinking, feelings, reactions, and interactions with their world.
- Understanding what to expect helps you anticipate, understand, and mold desirable behaviors sensitively.
- Every child is unique and should be treated as such.

Obstacles to Health and Well-Being

n a perfect world, raising kids is straightforward and easy. You have the knowledge you need, your child happily cooperates, and things progress swimmingly. No obstacles, no hiccups, no curveballs. But that's not reality. Real-life obstacles to your child's physical health and emotional well-being do exist. These threats can happen to any child, of any size. But for children with smaller and larger bodies, these challenges can be damaging to their health and well-being. I'm going to walk you through what I consider the most important challenges . . . so you're ready.

Interruptions in Body Functioning

The goal of physical health is a body that functions well. It does all the things it's supposed to do with ease. But how do you know if your child's body is functioning well? You must look beyond the BMI or a growth chart. When your child goes for an annual checkup, the doctor reviews their metabolic parameters, such as blood pressure and cholesterol, and their habits around movement, sleep, and eating. They will also review how your child is doing socially and at school. All these factors influence your child's physical functioning.

If you have a child who is larger or smaller, the amount of body fat they carry may or may not alter their body functioning. Too little body fat can impair body temperature control, for instance. A little bit of extra padding is unlikely to deter body functioning, while ample amounts may task the body and its systems. I won't dive into each of these potential conditions deeply, but I want you to have a sense of what they are should your health-care provider mention them.

- **High blood pressure (hypertension):** High blood pressure occurs mostly in older kids and can happen for different reasons, including too much body fat, a family history of hypertension, type 2 diabetes, high cholesterol, or exposure to secondhand smoke. Hypertension is more common in children who carry abundant body fat. However, it also occurs in children who are smaller and midsize.

- **High blood fats (hyperlipidemia):** Seven percent of US kids have high cholesterol, according to the CDC. High concentrations of lipids in the bloodstream change the way the body processes and regulates blood fats like cholesterol, triglycerides, and lipoproteins. Pediatricians routinely check blood cholesterol between ages nine and eleven, but may do so earlier, especially if your child carries more body fat or has a family history of high cholesterol.

- **High blood sugar (insulin resistance):** Insulin regulates the amount of sugar that floats in your child's bloodstream and keeps it in a normal range. But when a child has insulin resistance, sugar in the bloodstream builds up, also known as prediabetes. Prediabetes eventually leads to type 2 diabetes if untreated. The prevalence of both types of diabetes, type 1 and 2, in children aged six to nineteen has doubled from 2001 to 2017.

- **Nutrient deficiencies:** Any nutrient deficiency can complicate the physical health and body functioning of any child, potentially causing cognitive delays or fatigue, or interrupting bone development. A concern for all children is vitamin D, but especially for those with larger bodies. Studies show that vitamin D is overabsorbed by fat tissue and gets "sequestered," or trapped, making it unavailable in the bloodstream, placing children at very high risk for vitamin D deficiency. Smaller children can experience nutrient deficiencies that cause anemia and affect their skin, hair, and teeth, causing dry skin, hair loss, and cavities. Nutrient deficiencies can and do exist for kids of all sizes.

- **Bone health:** Children with diets deficient in calcium and vitamin D, and who aren't physically active, are at greater risk for poor bone health and an increased risk of bone fractures. Studies show a 25 percent increased risk of arm and leg fractures when the diet is deficient, and twice as much risk in larger-bodied children, most likely due to interruptions in nutrient availability, as explained above. Smaller children may have inadequate consumption of calcium and vitamin D, causing bone loss or poor bone growth.

- **Indigestion:** Anywhere from 10 to 25 percent of children complain of gastroesophageal reflux (GERD) symptoms on a weekly to monthly basis. Children who have more body fat tend to have more symptoms of GERD.

- **Other concerns:** Children with smaller bodies, or who are chronically underweight, may experience decreased heart rate, low blood pressure, and low body temperature. Constipation may occur due to slower movement of the gastrointestinal tract. Also, there may be long-term consequences on bone and heart health, including osteopenia (bone softening), osteoporosis (bone weakening), and poor circulation to the heart and lungs.

The Toll of Size Bias and Stigma

A significant challenge to supporting your child's emotional well-being are the societal norms around size. *Size bias* is the negative attitudes, beliefs, and stereotypes aimed at a child simply because of their size. For instance, the assumption that a child is ill or unhealthy based on their size is a common bias. Stigmatizing words like "obesity" or "failure to thrive" in the doctor's office, or using BMI Report Cards in schools, are examples of potentially stigmatizing situations that may undermine your child's worthiness. As a parent, you may experience assumptions about your parenting skills if you're raising a larger- or smaller-bodied child. Even a conversation

> **#TruthBomb:** Implicit bias, or the internal beliefs of which we are unaware, is common among parents, teachers, and health-care providers, especially about size.

with the doctor that opens with "Let's talk about your child's weight" may cause you shame and embarrassment, leaving you feeling like a failure.

Size stigma describes the discriminatory acts targeted against children because of their size. Most commonly, size stigma shows up as bullying. "Tommy won't change his clothes in the locker room before gym," said Sheila, mom of a thirteen-year-old boy who worried about his belly. "I don't get it. I think he's fine, but he's afraid he'll get teased, so he changes in the bathroom stall." In any child, but especially in children with larger or smaller bodies, bullying can lead to psychological problems, including anxiety, depression, and refusing to go to school.

Studies show that children who experience size discrimination have a lower quality of life. In children with larger bodies, size stigma sets the conditions for poor health outcomes, such as unhealthy eating

#WiseAdvice: Teach your child to appreciate and accept all bodies of every size, as early as possible (toddlerhood!).

behaviors, lower physical activity, substance abuse (in teens), body fat gain, depression, and low self-esteem. Furthermore, children and teens who've experienced size-based teasing may gain body fat and develop binge eating behaviors, weight fluctuations, and low self-esteem in adulthood. Children with smaller bodies experience size stigma, too. Bullying and teasing may lead to poor self-esteem, depression, poor academic performance, and isolation from peers. Of course, *any* discrimination against *any* child for *any* reason can have negative effects on their health and well-being.

Unfortunately, size stigma happens as early as toddlerhood and doesn't originate just from a child's peer group—it comes from educators, family members, and the media. Even doctors, nurses, and other health-care providers may be unconsciously biased against a child's size. Children who experience bias or stigma may experience significant

STIGMA + BIAS = BODY DISSATISFACTION

"I have a son of thirteen who is unhappy with his size," wrote Maeve. "He says his legs (thighs) are too big—he hates them—and wishes he could get surgery, which to be honest was a big shock and a bit of a shame to hear. It's upsetting that my boy would even put surgery and himself in the same sentence." Feeling unhappy about one's size, shape, or appearance is called body dissatisfaction, and it's on the rise, beginning at younger ages and including more boys than ever before. When a child is dissatisfied with their body, they are at higher risk for anxiety, depression, disordered eating, and eating disorders. I get it if you feel your stress hormones elevating as you read this. I'm with you. It seems impossible (and dangerous) to send your precious child out into the world, especially if their size varies from the "norm." But if you're going to instill emotional well-being in your child and be the support system they need, you'll need to model body acceptance and teach them as early as possible to be accepting of all sizes.

stress as a result, which may interfere with their emotional well-being and physical health.

Teach your child to appreciate and accept all bodies of every size, as early as possible (toddlerhood!). And remember, you can't unconditionally accept your child if you're bashing your own or others' food choices or body size. You can't "walk the talk" if you struggle to accept yourself, or others. This book offers you an opportunity to chart a new course. A chance to change your mindset and check your biases, so you can help your child grow up to be accepting of every body, including their own.

How to Support Your Whole Child

N ow that you understand the physical and emotional building blocks of health, you're ready to build the lifestyle habits that secure a future of health and well-being. But before we get there, I want to drive home two main concepts.

Focus on Function, Not Size

Your child's daily environment and the lifestyle habits they build can overrule their genetic predisposition for size and health. Of course, you can monitor what's happening with your child's physical health by using the tools we've covered here, but remember, there's more to the story than the number on the scale or percentile on the growth chart. Your child's physical functioning—how they move and regulate their daily functions—affects their health, too.

If your child has a health condition that impacts their physical functioning, concentrate on this, rather than on their size or body weight as the problem. Focusing too much on size contributes to shame and stigma, which may worsen physical health. Body function is *far more important* than your child's size. Optimal physical functioning at *every* size is the goal.

Navigate Stressors with Resilience

Resilience is your child's ability to handle stress like bias and stigma. What makes a child resilient? Healthy self-esteem and strong social support. Positive self-esteem moderates stress *internally*, allowing your child to use their developmental skills, like reasoning or self-efficacy (their past abilities to navigate stress), to work through it. Social support, like a caring adult, offers *external* ways to moderate stress, such as talking through a negative situation or offering physical comfort. Both buffer stress. All kids will face struggles, and these aren't always "bad." They allow for the development of self-regulation and adaptive skills, and offer an opportunity to teach coping skills.

Thankfully, scientists have teased out the factors that build resilient kids. Keep in mind, these vary based on your unique child and family unit, and where your child is in their development. Resilient kids have:

- Caring family members who are sensitive and nurturing
- Close, secure relationships and a sense of belonging within the family
- Skilled parents who are good at managing the family
- A sense of control and the motivation to cope and adapt to changes and disappointments
- Problem-solving skills, planning skills, and a family that is flexible
- An ability to regulate behavior and emotions
- A positive view of self and family
- Optimism and a positive family outlook
- A belief that life has meaning; a desire to make a meaningful life; a family with purpose
- Family routines and rituals
- A well-functioning school
- Connections with well-functioning communities

Chart a New Course

Cultivating the habits of health and well-being requires more than simply getting your child to eat their fruit and vegetables . . . though this simple message is all we hear. Although you may want this to be easy, it isn't. *But it can be easier.* Whether you're worried about your child or just want to learn how to build lifestyle habits for a future of health and well-being, my intent is to provide you with guidance, insight, and a path forward that meets you exactly where you are. My hope is to change how you experience and relate to your child, at every size and stage of development, so they can grow up healthy and happy.

Together, we'll chart a new course. I'll help you take charge of what you can—the environment your child is growing up in—and spearhead a new pathway focused on health-promoting behaviors. Next, you'll be introduced more fully to the 8 Pillars of Wellness. These represent the lifestyle habits and attitudes every child needs to grow up physically healthy *and* emotionally strong, at every size. Your child deserves a healthy, happy future, and you deserve to feel good about parenting your precious child!

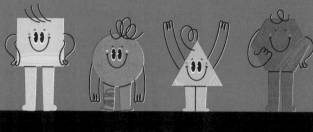

PART 2

The 8 Pillars of Wellness

You are born into your family and your family is born into you. No returns. No exchanges.

—**ELIZABETH BERG**

FAMILY CULTURE
All for One and One for All

The Garcia family eats together as often as they can. Both parents are active. He jogs and has a physically demanding job as a landscaper. She walks her dog and loves to garden. They like to take their three kids hiking on the weekends, or to the beach in the summer. Their kids range from five to nine years, and the older two are involved in after-school activities like Scouts and soccer. The family attends most events together, supporting each child in their activities. The Garcias understand their limits on time and energy and take care to be involved without overcommitting their resources. You could say they have figured out a way to balance their work and family demands, prioritizing what they call "together time," whether that's on the soccer field or with their spiritual congregation. They're cultivating a strong sense of family.

Although the Garcias might not know it, they're on to something. Studies show that children flourish when the connectedness of the "family," however it may be defined, is embedded within a network of friends, family, community, and congregations. By doing many things as a unit, in and outside of their home, the Garcias are weaving their family "fabric," something that will be hard to tear apart. Even parents who are divorced or separated can foster this connection when they provide love and security and co-parent collaboratively, putting the kids and family first.

As the first Pillar of Wellness, family culture is the cornerstone of your child's self-esteem, health behaviors, and sense of safety and belonging. It's where it all begins. A strong family culture is protective, while a weak one can undermine self-esteem, emotional well-being, and mental health. It's the sturdy support *every* child needs, especially if they have a larger or smaller body.

SCIENCE AND SOCIETY
The Ties That Bind

" I was brought up by a very strict mom—you must clean your plate before you get a dessert, candy stored up on the top shelf and used as a reward, or withheld as punishment," described Nicole. "Now I overeat and have this mindset that sweet stuff is on a pedestal and even find myself secretly eating chocolate and cookies." I've heard many stories like this over my career. You may have a similar story, whether it be about food and eating, exercise, or any other habit. Your habits and behaviors began in your family. Your attitudes, self-view, and worldview began there, too.

Your experiences in childhood live in you, and you bring them to your family. They're present in your attitudes, beliefs, and everyday actions, whether you're consciously aware of them or not. For instance, your family may have held strong opinions about food (*processed food is toxic*), certain body shapes or sizes (*round is unhealthy*), or exercise (*only intense exercise matters*). Some of these dogmas about nutrition, health, and exercise may be beneficial, while others may not be. What was learned in childhood may have led to a healthful lifestyle, or it may have left you with habits with which you struggle today. "I am one thousand percent conscious of my biases and experiences and don't want to pass them on to my daughter," Nicole said.

Raising a child with positive lifestyle behaviors calls on your role-modeling skills, how you think about yourself, and your ability to guide and govern a family. It requires a strong family culture that accepts, respects, and supports your child, no matter what.

The Family Bond: A Far-Reaching Influence

Family culture is the set of values, practices, ideas, and attitudes of the family. It's knitted within the home environment and family dynamic. From mealtimes, holiday gatherings, and community activities to the family's belief system, like the responsibility to give back to the community, the family "culture" is woven into the fabric of daily living and lifestyle behaviors. In essence, family culture is *who your family is as a family*. And it's the most important, influential ethos with which your child will grow up.

Strong family bonds not only encourage your child to become their best self, they also reduce the risk of negative outcomes, like substance abuse. In fact, for a child, the cornerstone to thriving and succeeding in life is the presence of a strong family bond. Family connection, acceptance, and nurturance in the home include five important areas: care, support, safety, respect, and participation. Additionally, children succeed when they have self-acceptance, purpose in life, positive relationships with others, personal growth, mastery of their environment, and autonomy. Children who have the greatest family connectedness are almost *50 percent more likely* to do well compared to children with the weakest family bonds.

The good news is strong family bonds may exist even when life serves up challenges like single parenting, food insecurity, poverty, or other circumstances beyond one's control that stress or run counter-culture to the traditional family structure. The idea that families need to have two parents and money for vacations and extracurricular activities for their children to thrive and have good outcomes simply isn't true. Children who feel loved by, connected to, cared for, and bonded with their caretaker are set up to flourish, regardless of the family circumstances.

> **#WiseAdvice:** When a family is connected, children *thrive* rather than simply survive.

Family culture primes the circuitry for how your child thinks, behaves, and feels about themself and others in the world. Prioritizing "family first" emphasizes a warm, close, supportive family tie over the individual, and has been associated with psychological health, including prosocial behavior like kindness toward others and well-being. The opposite—loose family ties, and a cold or unsupportive family environment—has the opposite effect, contributing to poor psychological and physical well-being, and antisocial behavior.

Think of family culture as a protective "bubble." Your child can see the world and what's happening—good and not so good—and learns about it from a protected, safe environment. Family culture binds and supports its members in good times and hard, and is a safe place where every child belongs, is accepted, and loved. It can also soften the impact and damage of peer pressure, stigma, bias, and exclusion, and imparts real-time guidance when your child responds to a negative comment, a bully, or a classmate who questions why they pack vegetables in their lunch box. It's the voice in their head asking, *What would my mom/dad/ family say or do?* when faced with a challenging situation or a difficult decision.

The Power of the Role Model

Coupled with a strong family bond, nothing is more impactful to a child than watching how their parent or caregiver moves through the world on a day-to-day basis. Simply watching what a parent does and how they think and react sets the blueprint for what is "normal behavior." From how you put on your makeup or shave; how you exercise, relax, and eat; to what you say about your body—these little everyday actions mold your child's attitudes and behaviors. Role modeling is a silent, powerful influence throughout childhood.

Parents with healthful behaviors, such as eating fruits and vegetables, being physically active, and maintaining steady health, have children who are ten times more likely to eat fruits and vegetables and be active, and three times more likely to be physically well. Ironically, what a parent eats is *less* important than modeling what healthy eating looks like. Witnessing healthful behaviors like shopping for nutritious foods or cooking at home has a favorable influence, improving children's overall diet quality, even if what is eaten isn't necessarily nutritious. And when you demonstrate enjoyment of eating and positive health behaviors, the influence on your child is quite positive, shaping their behaviors. And guess what? Family meals are the most influential on children's food choices and eating habits simply through the interactions around the table.

> **#TruthBomb:** From preschool to preteen, children are open and willing to follow your lead. Take advantage of this decade and model the behaviors you want to see in your kids.

Role modeling reaches beyond food to other lifestyle habits, too. Being physically active and encouraging movement can increase your child's overall activity level. And if you cut the time spent in front of the television, computer, and smartphone, your child's use of TV, gaming devices, and computers may decrease as well. It's clear. *Your* health behaviors influence your child's health behaviors.

CHARACTERISTICS OF A GOOD ROLE MODEL

1. **Willpower:** Maintains routines, even when obstacles occur.

2. **Confidence:** Sets goals for the whole family and pursues them.

3. **Flexibility:** Rolls with the ups and downs of unexpected changes, adapting behaviors to stay on track with family routines and goals.

4. **Respect:** Shows it for self and others; responds with understanding and empathy.

5. **Commitment:** Works to achieve goals despite failure, adversity, or setbacks.

6. **Self-improvement:** Desires growth and improvement as an individual and for the family unit.

7. **Honesty:** Owns mistakes and missteps. Encourages open communication of thoughts, opinions, and beliefs.

8. **Accountability:** Accepts mistakes and areas of growth; adjusts to maintain goals.

·············· **Takeaways:** ··············

- A strong family bond protects a child's physical and emotional health while a weak one may compromise them.

- Family culture not only imparts positive behaviors, but sets the tone for the attitudes, beliefs, and biases your child will take out into the world.

- Positive role modeling offers your child greater odds of absorbing healthful behaviors and habits—more than any words, discussion, or lesson can offer.

OBSTACLES AND OBJECTIONS
Bias and Parent Struggles

From a very young age, we teach our children things that stick with them for a lifetime. We parents frequently share in society's dichotomy of *bad* and *good*: Good grades and bad grades; good manners and bad manners; sweets are bad and vegetables are good; and good people and bad people are everywhere. In doing so, we accept these binaries as the norm even when they don't necessarily serve our children or ourselves. These messages become instilled deep within, shaping your child's worldview, and more important, how they see themself. Even if you've worked hard to plant values like social justice, equality, and acceptance, these may be challenged when your child heads out the door.

Our society doesn't accept and include everyone. We each have our biases, learned long ago as children. Bias against size, color, creed, politics, and more. If your child is different in any way—in size, hair or skin color, clothing choice, physical abilities, or food traditions—they may be subject to bias and discrimination outside of your home.

Implicit Biases—We All Have Them

Our brain makes automatic associations as a way to sort through all the information it is fed. We automatically associate our experiences and belief systems with an image we drum up in our minds. For example, think of the word "beach." If you live on the West Coast, this may drum up white, vast swaths of sand. If you're from Maine, it may conjure rocky coastlines. We do this with all things—people, too. This is called implicit bias. An implicit bias is *a belief or attitude that we are unaware we hold*. Implicit bias develops early and is shaped by our home environment, the media, and our outside world. As a parent, you come to the job with your own implicit biases, even though they may oppose what you consciously believe and think. For instance, you may say it doesn't matter what your child eats or does, but have a negative reaction when they eat ice cream, watch too much TV, or skip dinner. This is your implicit bias surfacing.

Implicit biases about race, gender, and ethnicity are common. Whether it's how genders, ethnic groups, and people of different sizes are depicted on TV or talked about at home, your child is affected by implicit bias every day. From this, they form their own biases along the way, shaping how they relate to others and how they feel about themself.

Many of us have implicit biases about size. The most prevalent ones are the idea that *thin equals healthy* and *large is unhealthy*. Sadly, bias produces more bias. Parents of children who have midsize bodies (or appear to be of a "healthy size") demonstrate size bias against children with larger bodies. If a parent is biased against a child who is larger or smaller, it's fair to expect their child will pick up on these attitudes and show bias against others. It's important to be aware of this because the impact is twofold: Children who experience size bias may experience negative repercussions on their mental and physical health. And, if you're raising a child with a midsize body who develops a negative bias about people in larger or smaller bodies, chances are they will perpetuate the cycle of bias and discrimination.

Size bias shows up in obvious and unexpected places. Children who name-call, degrade, or bully another child based on their size are demonstrating size bias and stigma. Teachers who make assumptions about the characteristics or abilities of a child based on their size,

> **#TruthBomb:** Children as young as three years old demonstrate size bias, and children aged nine to eleven years have an implicit bias against children of larger size to a magnitude similar to that of racial bias.

like being lazy, are doing the same. Benching children of various sizes in sports under the assumption of lesser physical abilities is yet another example. Less obvious are the ads and movies that depict larger-bodied individuals as inferior. Studies show teasing or criticizing *any* person about their size worsens their health. For children, size discrimination significantly worsens their quality of life. Imagine the impact of size bias when it happens in the home.

Size Discrimination in the Family System

"I was seven when I heard my mom talking to her friend about how much I weighed," shared Luanne, a mom. "I weighed ninety pounds, was big-boned, and the tallest in my class." The shame from this discussion stuck with her. She credits it as being part of the reason she developed an eating disorder at the age of twenty-one. Sadly, 37 percent of teenagers report weight-based teasing at home. Women in larger bodies recalled home as the *most significant source* of size stigma, with 53 percent reporting teasing or other forms of discrimination from their mothers and 44 percent reporting it from their fathers.

Unfortunately, the family environment isn't always a safe, nurturing place for children. Bullying can come from parents, siblings, and extended family members. Between siblings, this can include hitting, name-calling, and teasing. From parents, it's shaped by criticism, unequal treatment, and the use of unflattering words and characterizations. Treating your child differently based on their size, like creating separate meals or different rules for eating, can erode how a child feels about themselves. For instance, a parent might restrict second helpings or try to get a larger child to exercise more than others in the family. They may unintentionally use hurtful words to describe their child's size or behaviors, all of which can damage the family connection and the child's sense of self. For the child who is smaller, a parent may offer dessert every night but discourage exercise. Singling out one child from the rest of the family sends a strong message: the child is different. Although it may be necessary to treat a child as such, as in the case of diabetes or a food allergy, when the differential treatment is due to size, it can be damaging. There is nothing more alienating than feeling like you don't belong.

"We often share marginalized identities with other members of the family," says Dr. Kendrin Sonneville, a professor at the University

Instead of . . .	Do this . . .	Why
Body-shaming	Respect and listen to your child. Emphasize "All bodies are good bodies."	Teasing based on size may erode self-esteem and trust. People come in all sizes. Size discrimination is harmful.
Name-calling or using labels like "picky" or "fat" or "lazy"	Avoid using labels. Focus on inner qualities and characteristics.	Labels can be internalized and self-fulfilling, limiting a child's potential growth.
Ignoring or brushing off a child's concerns about body or size	Calm them with positivity, like "You are enough" or "You're doing a fine job." Don't disregard a concern that comes up often.	Disregarding worries can invalidate feelings, neglect an emotional challenge, and shut down conversation.
Pushing for perfection in eating, size, or other health-related efforts	Relay realistic messages like "Nobody is perfect," and "Imperfection is what makes a person interesting!"	Overvaluing perfection may diminish worthiness and confidence and lead to perfectionistic thinking.
Treating a larger or smaller child differently from the rest of the family	Treat everyone the same; don't limit sweets for one and push them for another. Expect everyone to participate in activities.	Singling out a child from the rest of the family sends a negative message.

of Michigan School of Public Health whose research focuses on the prevention of eating disorders and weight stigma. "If you're being teased, often there are people in your family with similar identities, creating comfort and safety, but if you're teased about the way your body looks by your family, the folks that are supposed to align with you and support you are the ones causing harm and that can be so destructive." Certainly, if the family culture is discriminating toward children with larger or smaller bodies, a child may have a harder time in the real world where size bias, stigma, and diet culture run rampant. In fact, research suggests the family dynamic is powerful when it comes to outside forms of bias and discrimination. A strong family culture and dynamic softens the blow of discrimination, but it's not enough to buffer the influence. However, a *negative* family culture compounds and worsens the effects of discrimination.

It never bodes well for a child to hear an adult commenting on the size of their body, whether it comes from a doctor, teacher, or their own family. *You're one strong kid* can build self-confidence, while *You're getting bigger* can undermine self-worth. But even a compliment may draw too much attention to appearance. Watch what you say about your child, others, and yourself. Kids may associate with the words they hear and assume these labels and attitudes.

There's no doubt that well-intentioned relatives and peers place pressure on the main caretaker, often the mother, about their child's

BODY-SHAMING

Body-shaming is the act of humiliating someone by mocking them or making negative comments about their body size or shape. It's a form of size stigma and can occur in families and outside the home. For larger individuals, it's referred to as "fat-shaming." For smaller people, it may be called "skinny-shaming." Many children, regardless of size, experience body-shaming. Maybe they've heard other kids teasing the "big kid" on the playground or shunning the "scrawny kid." Or perhaps they've heard adults talk of weight loss or weight gain diets. Children may even ask, "Am I fat?" or "Am I too skinny?" When parents participate in or align with body-shaming, it becomes normalized in the home. Unfortunately, this makes it too easy for children to internalize these biases—no matter their size—and experience the consequences, or persecute others, perpetuating the social norms of body bias and discrimination.

body size and eating behaviors. From grandparents telling grand-children "You have to take a bite of everything on your plate" to teachers calling out or commenting on a child's lunch box contents, these external forces place more pressure on you, despite you doing your best to raise a healthy child.

Remember, your attitudes about food, health, and, yes, size come from many factors. The family culture you grew up in is one of them. How you were treated and whether you were criticized about your weight, eating, or size may have given you the message that you weren't good enough. In order to be good enough, you may have learned you needed to shrink, eat differently, or bulk up. As such, you may have wounds from your childhood that haven't healed—and your own beliefs and attitudes about another person's appearance or behaviors reflect what you learned and experienced in childhood. To be a good role model and create a loving, supportive family culture, any lingering wounds must heal, and any inherent biases must be addressed.

A Struggle with Past Eating and Body Challenges

I once had a client—I'll call her Debbie—who had no kids. Puzzled when she arrived for her first appointment, I asked, "How can I help?" Debbie told me she had struggled with disordered eating and poor body image since she was a teen. She had a past of being in and out of treatment centers for an eating disorder, and at the age of twenty-seven, she felt she had overcome a condition that had dominated the last decade of her life. She was recently married and she and her husband were talking about starting a family. "I want to make sure I don't 'give' my child an eating disorder," said Debbie. "How can I prevent my eating disorder from transferring to my child?" Debbie's self-awareness of her past struggles and how they might affect her future children was impressive.

As parents, *we all come to the table with our stuff*—our past eating experiences, body image, self-esteem, and other psychological strug-gles. And we risk transferring some of this stuff on to our kids. Studies show that children whose mothers had a past history of an eating disorder had a higher risk of developing one themselves. But if you've struggled with your own body and eating demons in the past, it doesn't mean your child will. Protective factors include having a healthy family environment around food, including frequent family meals, a positive mealtime vibe, and avoiding "body and eating talk" at the table.

Of course, the family culture proves powerful here, too. High-quality family relationships, including connectedness and good family functioning, are protective against disordered eating behaviors. Importantly, when parents and extended family members don't influence children to lose weight or meet societal norms of thinness, kids are more protected against disordered eating and body dissatisfaction and are buffered against cultural pressures around size and appearance.

#WiseAdvice:
I encourage you to explore your own food, body, and eating history. Poor self-esteem, dieting, and self-sabotaging comments are red flags that may unintentionally affect your child's emotional health and your family culture.

You don't need to have had an eating disorder to transfer your own eating, food, and body issues to your child. Remember, you're a role model and the gatekeeper of family culture. Dieting and especially talking about food and weight may lead to negative eating behaviors in children. The point of understanding your own current or past struggles (and those of your partner if you have one) is that you can actively work through these issues and prevent them from becoming your child's struggles. While you don't necessarily need to make an appointment with a dietitian or psychotherapist like Debbie did, this can be a valuable strategy for changing your mindset, healing past experiences, improving your interactions with your child, and ultimately protecting them from the risks associated with your past.

You're the most powerful agent in cultivating a strong, supportive family culture and promoting body acceptance. By checking your own biases, making a conscious effort to break negative cycles, and healing childhood wounds, you can mitigate the biases that may harm your child and others.

- Your child's worldview and self-view are a reflection of the family culture and may be challenged by the real world.

- Bias and discrimination may happen within the home, school, health-care system, and outside world. A strong, supportive family culture can soften any potential negative impact.

- A parent may have insecurities and unhealed wounds from childhood that may make it challenging for them to strengthen the family culture and raise a child with body confidence.

HOW TO STRIVE AND THRIVE
Cultivate Your Family Culture

Every child (and parent and family) deserves to be respected, accepted, and included, no matter their size. So how do you actually create a strong family culture, and cultivate a climate of unconditional acceptance so your child can stand confident in themself? Of course, there are lots of things to consider, but I've boiled this down to four areas: creating a body-neutral home; optimizing your role as a model of health and well-being; striving for acceptance, inclusion, and dignity; and optimizing your family functioning. Let's dig in!

A Body-Neutral Home

When it comes to size and our children, our own attitudes, actions, and language matter. In other words, you need to understand whether you are negative, positive, or neutral about bodies, as it will come out in your words and actions. Body negativity is a negative view of the body. It focuses on deficits or imperfections. *Your legs are too skinny. Your tummy is always so bloated. I wish your hair wasn't so straight (or curly).* Body positivity is the opposite—an appreciative view of the body, regardless of shape, size, or other appearance factors. *Your body is beautiful just the way it is.* Last, body neutrality takes the focus off of appearance altogether and places it on body function or abilities, centering on what the body can do with no attachment to what it looks like.

There are no benefits to body negativity, especially when it comes to children. But there are benefits to being both body-positive and body-neutral. Both aim to break the link between the body and worthiness, emphasizing dignity, respect, and fairness, no matter one's size. But there's no denying that one—body positivity—does center on how one looks. And for some children this will be too much focus on appearance, as some will still struggle with accepting how they look. That's where body neutrality comes in. It doesn't worry about appearance. Its focus is on inner qualities and function, not form. *Your legs can take a long walk. Your arms can swing a tennis racket. Your body is flexible. You easily connect with others.* (For kids with physical disabilities or differences, the messages can be even more pointed.) Body neutrality is a move toward accepting the body your child (and you!) has. Here are a few tips for cultivating a body-neutral home:

Focus on signature strengths. Your child has something they're good at or an admirable quality. Maybe they're a good writer. A loyal friend. A natural at sports, music, or drama. A math wiz. A kid who can figure things out. Emphasize these over any appearance element. From an early age (and thanks to my mother-in-law), I told all of my kids they were "strong and powerful." When strangers or other adults commented on their appearance, I redirected or replied with "She's really funny." "He's empathetic toward others," "She's got a great work ethic." You, too, can avoid mentioning how someone looks, and instead comment on personal qualities, abilities, and internal characteristics, such as funny, loyal, quick-witted, empathetic, sensitive, practical, diplomatic, athletic, or graceful. Use these inner quality descriptors to talk about yourself, too! Remember, telling your child they're beautiful every day emphasizes their appearance and may undermine their self-worth. Make sure you emphasize qualities and character over appearance.

Moderate the critic. Negative feedback can instill shame. Criticism is counterproductive to your child feeling good about themself. Equally as important is how you talk about yourself, and how you talk to and about your child, as it may become your child's internal dialogue. Instead of "Don't post that picture—I have a double chin," you could say, "I love that you caught me laughing here—that's such a happy picture of me!" Instead of "These pants make me look fat," you could say, "I'm not in love with these pants anymore." And avoid comments like "I've had too much to eat—back on my diet tomorrow!" Instead say, "Gosh, I really

SELF-COMPASSION AND ACCEPTANCE

If you've succumbed to the pressures and norms of society, take time to reflect on how this may be affecting your feelings and parenting. Show yourself compassion. Self-compassion replaces the judgment and critical evaluations we make of ourselves. Instead of focusing on shortcomings or failures, self-compassion allows you to be empathetic and compassionate to yourself, which then extends to others, according to Dr. Kristin Neff, founder of the Center for Mindful Self-Compassion. She outlines three elements of self-compassion: self-kindness versus self-judgment, common humanity versus isolation, and mindfulness versus overidentification. In self-kindness versus self-judgment, the focus is on the understanding that we are not perfect. Failure, imperfection, and falling short are inevitable. Knowing this, Dr. Neff encourages us to take the path of self-kindness, rather than fight against imperfection with frustration, self-criticism, and anger. The second element, common humanity versus isolation, reminds us that we all suffer. You aren't the only one who suffers. Last, to be in emotional balance, we must acknowledge our negative feelings with clarity and openness and not deny them. She points out that we cannot ignore our feelings *and* show compassion at the same time. Nor do we want to become caught up in negativity. Self-compassion can keep you emotionally balanced, aiding you through shortcomings, disappointment, and guilt. "A newborn baby is intrinsically worthy of care and warmth and kindness," Dr. Neff reminds us. "So are we as human beings."

enjoyed that meal!" Remember, you are only one influence in your child's life, but your consistent, repetitive acceptance of yourself and your child will plant seeds of self-acceptance.

Support through challenges. Your child will come up against challenging situations that call into question their worthiness, no matter their size. If your child is expressing concern or dissatisfaction about their body, sit down and have a conversation about how the feelings we have about our bodies can fluctuate. One day we may feel strong and confident, and on another day, anxious and depressed. It's a normal part of the human experience. It's okay to acknowledge that nobody feels 100 percent good, confident, and positive all the time. But don't dwell on bad feelings. Focus on the positive things, and try to find ways to highlight your child's positive qualities regularly.

If your child experiences teasing by family members or bullying by peers, stand up for them. Be the Mama or Papa Bear. Say something. Your child will see you love them, accept them, and act on their behalf. Educate others if need be. Say things like "We appreciate and accept all bodies." Having supportive and sensitive conversations with your child can help them get through confusing and hurtful situations feeling loved and important.

Be a Great Role Model

What is good for your child is also good for you! As you move through the Pillars of Wellness, let them guide you toward the habits you may need to refine or even put into place for yourself. Ask yourself, *Am I walking the talk? Am I "doing" instead of "telling"?* This will help you stay on track with what you desire for your child, habit-wise.

Your words *and* your actions matter. Remember, "good versus bad" is a binary attitude. Explore more open language. For instance, there are all kinds of food, yet we tend to describe them in black-and-white terms. I encourage you to avoid dualistic categorizations. Try to describe food more specifically or objectively, such as *[Food] is energizing for the body, satisfying to the appetite, appealing to the eye (and tummy), nourishing to the body, good for brain focus, supports strong muscles, or encourages the body to grow.* There are lots of ways to talk about food, eating, and

How to Handle Tricky Body-Shaming Scenarios

Scenario	What you can say	How it helps
Your child has been body-shamed at school.	"Teasing or bullying is not okay, especially when it's about how you look. This is body-shaming and I know it hurts. I hope you know that I think you are so much more! You're [fill in with qualities, abilities, characteristics]. These are what really matter. How are you feeling? Let's figure out how to handle this in the future."	Acknowledges the pain associated with bullying. Calls out discrimination— puts a name to it so your child can call it out. Emphasizes inner qualities. Prioritizes this as a problem that needs a solution.
One sibling teases another, using body size as ammunition.	**To the teaser:** "We don't put each other down in this family. It's wrong to bully anyone based on what they look like, especially your [sibling]. How were you feeling in that moment? Let's think of a different way to handle your feelings." Or simply say: "Mind your own body." **To the teased:** "I'm sorry [sibling] teased you. I know that hurts. Teasing is not okay in this family. I've talked with [sibling] and they were feeling [emotion], which made them act that way. They know it's not okay. How are you feeling? How can I support you? When you're up to it, let's sit down together with [sibling] and sort this out."	Clarifies stance on teasing/ bullying within the family. Asks open, reflective questions of each child. Supports both. Encourages repair.

(Chart continues on next page.)

(Continued from previous page)

Scenario	What you can say	How it helps
Another adult comments on your child's body size (and calls into question your parenting).	"Raising kids is one of the hardest things I've done. There's a lot of pressure to be a certain size and look a certain way. But I know that what a person looks like on the outside is not who they are on the inside. I'm raising my child to love themself for who they are, and to show respect for others in the same way."	Acknowledges how difficult parenting is today. Places emphasis on personal characteristics not appearance. Drives home respect for all.
Your child asks, *Am I fat?* or *Am I too thin?*	"We all have different body shapes and sizes. It's what makes the world we live in more interesting. Your body does so much and it doesn't stop you from doing the things you enjoy, like [activity]. What can your body do?"	Emphasizes that differences are okay and to be celebrated. Asks the child to reflect on their strengths and abilities.

health habits without shaming. The goal is to help your child learn and develop an open, unbiased attitude.

Family meals are the perfect setting for role modeling. Of course, teaching manners is the obvious angle, but talking about food, health, and nutrition is the elephant at the table. Are you talking about food, your child's eating behaviors, and their effect on their health? Many families, in my experience, err on the side of too much "table talk," like Lin. She used the family meal to teach her children about nutrition and what to eat for their health. Her conversations centered on what was good, what was bad, and how to be healthier. She saw mealtime as a time to teach but didn't realize her emphasis on food and healthy eating was a turn-off and counterproductive. Instead, I encouraged Lin to show enjoyment in eating and have conversations about what's happening in her children's world, share "grins and grimaces" from their day, and allow each child at the table to take center stage on a topic of their choice. What matters most is togetherness and joy at the table.

An Environment of Acceptance, Inclusion, and Dignity

Your child needs to *feel* they're loved. Some kids will need overt reassurances and more obvious signs of love and acceptance. Don't be shy about telling your child how fabulous they are—your home might be the only place they hear this. Beyond that, create traditions, holiday routines, weekend plans, and activities your whole family can enjoy together. Togetherness reinforces inclusion and acceptance.

Body dignity is the expectation of respect and care for bodies of every size. While you want your child to learn to appreciate themself and care for their body, over time the goal is for them to learn to *expect* respect, inclusion, and equity—no matter their size. This is far different from what many people with larger or smaller bodies experience today. Hop on an airplane and you will find seats that are too small to accommodate every body size. The reality is we have a variety of body sizes in our world, and our lived environment doesn't always accommodate this fact. The world needs to catch up to size diversity. Children who grow up with body dignity will demand and advocate for changes that respect and include bodies of all sizes.

> **#WiseAdvice:** Food and body-centric table talk can sensitize a child in two ways: by alerting them to their inadequacies (making them feel bad) or by turning them off (demotivating them).

Not only do I encourage you to become skeptical and critical of social "norms," such as diet culture, thin idealism, and the exclusions in our common environments, but I urge you to reject harmful influences on your child and the family culture for which you are striving. Be an advocate for the acceptance, inclusion, and dignity of *every* body. It will send a strong and clear message to your child, planting the seeds of compassion, empathy, and humanity toward all.

Family Functioning: Manifesto, Meetings, and a Mantra

I liken running a family to running a business. Because I do both, it makes sense to me. A business has a mission—a "why we do what we do" statement—and a vision—a "where we are going" goal. A business has systems and strategies, growth plans, and regular checkpoints. To cultivate a strong family culture, you want to have a mission and a vision. I call this your family manifesto. This provides grounding and a unifying point for all family members. To support the mission and vision of your family, you'll want to have periodic family meetings. These help you reset when you need to, announce changes, discuss challenges, and get input from all members of the family. Of course, as the parent or caregiver, you are the leader.

The Family Manifesto

A manifesto is defined as a declaration of policy and aims. In other words, the "who we are and what we believe" family creed. Really, you can include just about anything in your manifesto, but I encourage you to think about what you believe and what you're trying to achieve when it comes to your family's health, well-being, and core values about body acceptance and diversity.

First, brainstorm what you want to include, such as your health values, core beliefs, and how you want everyone to treat each other. Discuss this with your parenting partner and children if they're old enough to participate. Create a family manifesto document. Get as creative with this as you like! Place the manifesto where everyone can see it. Update it as your family changes and grows.

You will use your family manifesto as a basis for creating a family mantra, or a saying that describes and grounds your family, reminding them of who they are. For my family, we use the term *Family Castle*. Simple enough, but it means so much more. When used in context, it refers to what we believe, how we show up and interact, and our sacred community. Powerful, family-unifying stuff. Your mantra can be as simple as your last name, or it can be a word or phrase that carries meaning and reflects the important aspects of your manifesto.

A FAMILY MANIFESTO EXAMPLE

"In Our House We . . ."

- Believe all bodies are good bodies.
- Appreciate everything our bodies can do.
- Understand that differences are what make people unique and interesting.
- Respect everyone, no matter their age, gender, color, creed, or size.
- Help support and champion each other.
- Enjoy eating a variety of foods for nourishment and pleasure; there are no "bad" foods.
- Try new foods and food experiences.
- Move every day because it makes us feel good in our mind, body, and soul.
- Get plenty of sleep to energize our mood, body, and ability to learn.
- Love each other no matter what.
- Apologize before bedtime for our mistakes, misdoings, and wrong words.
- Gather for family meals to connect as a family.
- Value kindness to all humans and creatures.
- Laugh and play as much as possible.

The Family Meeting

A business will schedule lots of meetings to check in on people, projects, and growth. While you don't need to have a weekly family meeting (though you can if you want to), periodically touching base as a family can help address concerns and future changes. Make family meetings positive gatherings where open, respectful communication is encouraged. They should be upbeat, inclusive of all opinions, and productive. You can have a family meeting about anything, such as where you want to take your next vacation, the distribution of chores, the celebration of an achievement, revising the family manifesto, or reviewing family schedules. Avoid taking over or talking at your child. Remember, family meetings are meant to be cooperative, not top-down or parent-centered. They're family-building activities designed to encourage communication, cohesiveness, and unity.

THE WHOLE-CHILD CHECKUP
Your Family Culture

Now that you've learned about family culture, let's check in on how you're doing. Wherever you find yourself, there's likely some work to do. Let's help you get started. First, identify where you're at right now: Learner, Striver, or Thriver.

The Learner: Where Do I Begin?

If you find you're a Learner, focus on the easy thing first: body talk. Less is more. Always. The mere focus on bodies—good or negative—can be problematic. Remember, your child thinks you're the best thing since Goldfish! Let that impression remain for as long as possible. Create an environment where only neutral or positive body talk is allowed—infrequently at that—and you'll have a strong first step in creating a body-appreciative home.

Then, inventory your role-modeling skills. Where do you excel? Maybe it's your exercise routine or your sleep habits. Awesome! Where do you need more work? Be honest with yourself. If you're sneaking chocolate at night like Nicole, then this is an area to work on. Reflect on why this behavior exists and address it (Pillar Five will help). You want to be a good example to your child in all areas of well-being and health. Nailing your role-modeling skills will make raising a child who is healthy and feels good about themselves a lot easier.

You may wonder why I haven't mentioned family functioning yet. While you could create a family manifesto and have family meetings right away, they may ring hollow if you're struggling with role-modeling skills. That said, you are free to address the elements of family culture in

Family Culture: Learner, Striver, or Thriver

	Learner	Striver	Thriver
A body-neutral home; acceptance, inclusion, and dignity	Dieting, negative body talk, and criticism are part of the daily home environment. Parents and/or kids may be struggling with body image. Child is treated differently from the rest of the family based on size. Teasing and other size-discriminatory acts occur.	Inconsistent with body talk about self and others; shifting the conversation to internal qualities. The whole family participates in positive lifestyle behaviors; hints of size bias may still exist. Child may or may not struggle with insecurity.	No negative body talk in the home; embraces and cultivates respect for all bodies. Size bias is not tolerated. Child feels loved, protected, and supported.
Role modeling	Parent struggles with positive health behaviors; may have unaddressed past eating and body image concerns.	Parent has some good health behaviors and is actively working on others. Doing things together as a family more often.	Parent embodies a health-promoting lifestyle. Refrains from talking too much about health and lifestyle, but models it instead.
Family functioning	Family does not have established routines for communication and connection like family meals, a manifesto, or meetings.	A manifesto is emerging or in place. Pursuing a supportive family dynamic, open communication, and family unity.	Methods to communicate, a manifesto, and parameters around what it means to be in your family are well established. Child is secure and identifies with the family unit.

the manner that suits you and your family best. Dare to be inspirational with your manifesto, even if what you write down feels out of reach. You'll have something to work toward and a reminder of the intended journey on which you're taking your family.

Always work on acceptance, inclusion, and dignity. Acceptance and inclusion may happen naturally as you create more "together time." Body dignity may be harder to wrap your arms around, especially if you're working on yourself. Don't worry. You can navigate body dignity alongside your child. With self-care and self-compassion, you can show your child they have a right to equal and fair treatment no matter their size.

The Striver: Let's Level Up

As a Striver, you're on the right path—and that's good news! Where can you tweak things further? Keep shifting the conversation to internal qualities and neutralizing body language. If you have family values in your head, like spending more time together, take action. Add these to your family manifesto or introduce these topics at mealtime or family meetings. Add in another family tradition. My kids are in their twenties, and we just added hiking on Thanksgiving afternoon (yes, in the freezing cold New England weather!). There's no limit to building new traditions and ways to further connect. If you're on the right path, take the next steps to deepen the connectedness of your family unit.

The Thriver: Keep Up the Good Work

Mastering family culture is a long game and something that should be nurtured and cared for over time. Every effort toward creating a family culture of acceptance, inclusion, togetherness, support, understanding, communication, respect, and fun is invaluable to your child's physical health and emotional well-being. Not only will your child benefit today, but you'll set the blueprint for your future generations.

*Sleep is the single most effective thing we can do
to reset our brain and body health each day.*

—MATTHEW WALKER

SLEEP
The Bedrock of Health

ow did you sleep? It's a question that comes out of my mouth almost every day, whether directed to my spouse, my children, or any visitor who happens to be in my home. I'm not obsessed with sleep, but it's pretty important to me. Over the years, I've come to recognize that a good night's sleep anchors my mood, focus, and sense of motivation and well-being. Believe me, it's not lost on me that this book has been written almost entirely in the early morning hours when I'm well-rested and my mind is clear.

In the last decade or two, sleep has become one of the most studied and discussed health habits on the planet. Why wouldn't you want to take advantage of a daily habit that improves memory and learning, spurs creativity, lowers food cravings, and wards off the common cold— even cancer—all while improving mood, happiness, and stress? Sleep has been connected to just about every desirable health outcome one could ever want. Yet it's elusive for many, including children.

Nearly half of US kids *don't* get enough sleep. Instilling sleep hygiene, or the environment and routines that encourage uninterrupted and adequate amounts of sleep, is one of the best investments you can make for your child's future health and well-being.

Refresh the Body and Mind

Have you ever taken a nap, and upon waking, felt incapacitated? As if your legs and arms were paralyzed and the initial movement was an effort? Or felt that first deep breath was surprisingly laborious? If you've transferred your sleeping child from the car to bed, you've experienced the lifelessness associated with deep sleep. In reality, though, all you can assess is the number of hours your child spent in bed and whether or not they're refreshed when they wake up. If your child is in a bad mood or their behavior has been more challenging than usual, you may say things like *You need a nap today*, or *Wow, you didn't get enough sleep last night—it's early to bed tonight.*

We often attribute our children's behavior and mood to whether they got a good night's sleep, and rightfully so. "The average person will spend a third of their life asleep and kids will spend even more of their life sleeping," says Dr. Cara Palmer, director of the Sleep and Development Lab at Montana State University. "We've known how important sleep is for physical health, but we are learning more and more about how important it is to psychological health." It turns out, getting quality sleep is much harder than simply logging enough time in bed.

Some kids will lie in bed for long periods before they fall asleep, especially if they have access to electronic devices. Ten hours in bed

Age	Recommended Hours of Sleep
3 to 5 years	10 to 13 hours (including naps)
6 to 12 years	9 to 12 hours
13 to 18 years	8 to 10 hours

might be only six or seven hours of sleep. As such, sleep research is shifting its focus from the total hours of sleep per night to the quality of sleep and the variability that happens from night to night. Although shorter sleep duration doesn't necessarily equal adverse outcomes for a child, the general consensus is that poor sleep has negative repercussions on health and emotional well-being.

Sleep is the workhorse of repairing the body, processing emotions, and solidifying the knowledge gained from the wakeful hours of living. It allows the brain and body to literally rejuvenate overnight. For children, sleep is also critical to their normal growth and development.

#TruthBomb: Nearly two-thirds of middle schoolers do not get enough sleep on school nights. Late bedtimes and early school start times limit their sleep. The American Academy of Pediatrics (AAP) and the American Academy of Sleep Medicine (AASM) recommend middle schoolers start school no earlier than 8:30 a.m. to improve sleep quality.

SHOULD MY CHILD TAKE MELATONIN?

M elatonin is naturally produced in the brain by the pineal gland and is released at night to tell the body it's time to go to sleep. Over-the-counter melatonin may be used to help children get to sleep while establishing better sleep habits, or to reset sleep schedules in older children and teens. Sometimes melatonin is used for children with ADHD and autism. Melatonin is not regulated by the Food and Drug Administration (FDA). Unfortunately, over the last decade incidences of melatonin poisoning have increased. Specific dosing guidelines for children don't exist to date. Plus, melatonin products may contain varying levels and additional substances—all of which aren't easy to decipher. Short-term use is considered safe, but melatonin's long-term effects on growth and health are unknown. If you're thinking about using melatonin for your child, discuss this thoroughly with your health-care provider first.

So how do you know if your child is getting a good night's rest? The National Sleep Foundation and other experts have outlined a variety of parameters indicating good quality sleep in children. It depends on the total hours of sleep, the amount of time it takes to fall asleep, whether there are disturbances in the night, and more. "A lot of parents aren't necessarily aware of how well their kids are sleeping," says Dr. Palmer. "They know they're in bed for the night and for the recommended amount of time, but the child's daytime behaviors, like struggles with emotions, attention, behavior, or challenges in school, can alert parents to take a closer look at their sleep." Some parameters of quality sleep include:

- The amount of time it takes your child to transition from being awake to being asleep. The transition should take between sixteen and thirty minutes. More than forty-five minutes contributes to poor sleep quality.

- The ratio of total time spent asleep versus the total time in bed, known as sleep efficiency (SE). If your child sleeps for seven hours but was in bed for eight hours, their SE would be about 87 percent (seven divided by eight). A child with less than 74 percent SE is thought to have poor sleep.

- Occurrences leading to physical arousal, such as dreams, sleepwalking, or sleep apnea before or during sleep, or external factors like TV or electronic devices. Frequent disturbances negatively affect sleep quality.

SLEEP DURING PUBERTY

You may notice your middle schooler or early teen is becoming a night owl, going to bed later and later—and becoming more and more sleepy during the day. There's a good reason for this! As kids enter puberty, their circadian rhythm naturally shifts, causing them to go to sleep later and wake up later, by about two hours. As a result, the average teen cannot get to sleep before 10:00 or 11:00 p.m., which affects their ability to wake up in the morning. About 70 percent of preteens and teens don't get enough sleep, logging less than eight hours a night.

- Spontaneous awakenings after falling asleep. One or fewer awakenings are considered as good sleep quality in children, and four or more are defined poor quality. If your child wakes up at night and is awake for more than forty-one minutes, it's also a sign of poor sleep quality.

The Benefits of a Good Night's Sleep

Sleep affects many health outcomes. Some parents will be inspired by the better mood and behavior aspect, while others may focus on the impact of sleep on academic performance or appetite regulation. The good news is this: a good night's sleep will increase the likelihood that your child will experience positive outcomes in their overall health and well-being. From intelligence and mental health to growth and appetite regulation, sleep is foundational. And it's a powerful ally in raising a healthy, happy child. Let's take a brief tour of what we know about the effects of sleep on children's health and emotional well-being.

Intelligence

Does sleep make your child smarter? There's a body of evidence linking sleep to cognitive development and performance in the classroom. For example, children who get adequate sleep seem to have better short-term memory, working memory, and math scores, and can efficiently split their attention in the classroom compared to children who get *one hour less sleep* per night during the school week.

Mental Health

Sleep is increasingly linked to mental health outcomes. Children with longer sleep duration have better moods and emotional regulation, and fewer psychological symptoms such as anxiety and depression. Lack of sleep may disturb emotional processing and significantly interfere with emotional regulation and reactivity.

Poor sleep may also worsen things for the child with anxiety. For instance, studies show kids with anxiety are more vulnerable to sleep difficulties, including disturbances, night awakenings, and loss of sleep. Inadequate sleep may make them more anxious and emotionally reactive, and create a negative disposition (having more negative emotions than positive ones). Even a child's quality of life may be impaired by a lack of sleep. In a study of three- to ten-year-olds who weren't able to maintain good sleep, more negative feelings about peer relationships and school lowered their overall quality of life.

Growth

Sleep is incredibly important to optimal physical development in children. Growth and development mostly happen when your child is sleeping. Sleep is required for cellular regeneration, the communication circuitry in the brain, and metabolic processes like blood sugar regulation. Sleep also enables the release of growth hormone, which stimulates nearly all growth in the body, including height, tissues, organs, and bones. Growth hormone is made in the pituitary gland, a small gland located between the left and right lobes of the brain, and is released in a pulse-like fashion throughout the day, but especially at night during deep sleep. The daily amount of growth hormone secreted increases as your child ages and is especially high during puberty when growth, especially height, takes off. Children who don't get enough sleep may have suppressed growth hormone secretion, leading to disruptions in their growth.

Some children may be more susceptible to gaining body fat when they don't get enough sleep. Longitudinal studies, or studies that observe children over a long period of time, conclude there's a link between short sleep duration (less than ten hours of sleep for children aged three to five years; less than nine hours for children aged six to twelve years; and less than eight hours for teens aged thirteen and older) and body fat. Additionally, between birth and four years, short sleep duration (less than twelve hours in infants and less than eleven hours in young toddlers) is associated with more body fat, as well as poor emotional regulation, impaired growth, more screen time, and higher risk of injury. Overall, research suggests that a shorter duration of sleep (compared to what is needed) is linked to higher body fat in infancy (40 percent more likely), early childhood (57 percent more likely), middle childhood (more than twice as likely), and adolescence (30 percent more likely).

So does more sleep help? Some research suggests that every additional hour of sleep may reduce the likelihood of gaining body fat. Take caution here, though. The focus should be on optimal sleep duration and quality of sleep for your child's age. Too much sleep may result in more sedentary behavior and less physical activity.

Appetite Regulation

Sleep also appears to have an influence on appetite. Leptin, which you'll learn more about in Pillar Five, is a hormone that signals fullness or satisfaction after eating. When there is sleep deprivation, leptin decreases, dulling the sensation of fullness. Ghrelin, the hormone that tells your child they're hungry, increases when sleep is lacking, causing more hunger. When sleep-wake patterns are disturbed, appetite hormones may be disrupted, potentially disturbing your child's eating and food choices.

Interestingly, poor sleep may change how your child thinks about food, too, viewing it as a positive reward and increasing their vulnerability for overeating. Preschoolers who missed a nap and had a later bedtime for one day had an increased appetite for higher-calorie foods. Specifically, they ate 21 percent more calories, 25 percent more sugar, and 26 percent more carbohydrates on the day of sleep loss and this persisted through the next day.

> **#TruthBomb:** A lack of sleep may make your child hungrier and less aware of their fullness after eating.

Although appetite regulation is influenced by many factors, the influence of sleep is gaining more attention, especially as it impacts children and their appetite, food choices, and growth.

Cardiovascular Health

High blood pressure, elevated blood fats, and extra body fat may shorten sleep duration and cause poorer quality sleep. When looking at the influence of sleep on heart health, blood pressure, and lipids, recent studies in children have shown that more sleep plus moderate physical activity are most favorable to their cardiovascular health.

The Sleep Effect on Health and Well-Being

	A Good Night's Sleep . . .	Health and Well-Being Outcomes
Brain and Cognitive Function	Allows brain circuitry to process and organize input from the day.	Better memory (both short- and long-term), higher math scores, greater intellectual capacity, better executive functioning, stronger ability to focus on more than one thing.
Growth	Promotes normal growth hormone secretion.	Optimal linear growth occurs. Repairs and regenerates cells, muscles, and organs.
Emotional Regulation	Encourages emotional processing.	Dreams help process emotions, creating positive effects on mood, behavior, and mental health.
Body Fat	Regulates appetite hormones and insulin.	May minimize swings in appetite, reduce overeating, and promote better food choices.
Cardiovascular System	Slows down heart rate and blood pressure, which allows body to rest and repair.	Improved cardiometabolic function.

·················· Takeaways: ··················

- Sleep is a powerful health habit, helping your child grow, learn, remember, and manage stress, emotions, and mood.

- Quality sleep is more important than the number of hours spent in bed.

- Lack of sleep can have widespread repercussions on physical health and emotional well-being.

OBSTACLES AND OBJECTIONS
Why Kids Don't Get Enough Sleep

Unfortunately, sleep disturbances in children are common. In fact, a third of children from infancy to age seventeen don't get the recommended amount of sleep for their age. Two-thirds of middle schoolers don't get enough sleep; and children of racial and ethnic minority groups, children who grow up with financial and social stress, and children who have special health-care needs are at even higher risk for inadequate sleep.

Abby, a past client of mine with attention-deficit/hyperactivity disorder (ADHD), struggled with restless legs syndrome (RLS), a sleep disorder and condition that affects 1.5 million children and adolescents. The primary symptom of RLS is an uncontrollable urge to move the legs. To relieve this impulse, children move their legs, stretch, get up and down, or toss and turn in bed. One reason for RLS is iron deficiency, but there are other culprits, like a genetic tendency or a neurologic condition. Abby was smaller and had low iron intake and iron deficiency. She was tired at school, had low energy levels, and was inattentive in the classroom. Eventually, her mood and behavior were affected. Improving her eating pattern and iron status improved her overall nutrition and growth, relieved her RLS symptoms, and improved her sleep, which started a cascade of quality-of-life improvements.

There are many things that can interrupt a good night's sleep. You need to understand these barriers so you can tackle them. Although they may not be an issue for you now, the trends indicate that sleep problems emerge as kids get older.

Willy-Nilly Bedtime Routines

Children thrive with structure, especially during the first decade of life. While predictable bedtime routines are a proven supporter of good sleep, many children don't have this experience. For example, if bedtime is at 7:00 p.m. one night, and the next it's 9:00 p.m., and it varies from night to night, or your child stays up later and sleeps in on the weekends, they may experience inadequate or poor quality sleep. Exciting activities before bedtime, like roughhousing or games of chase, can also make it difficult for your child to settle down and go to sleep. Unpredictability around bedtime can spark insecurity, which can affect your child's sleep, too.

Child Resistance

Of course, it's up to caregivers to set the environment for a good night's sleep, but children are a real factor, too. They may resist or try to delay their bedtime. To delay bedtime, young kids commonly get out of bed with questions, requests for a drink, or complaints of hunger. Older kids may stay up to catch up with peers, extend their studies, or unwind with a gaming device or television. Typically, the younger the child, the more they resist bedtime, and the more trouble they have sleeping through the night. But as kids get older, they report more difficulties with falling asleep. All told, these problems delay or interfere with sleep, compromising quality.

Screens and Artificial Light

Light triggers the brain to wake up. Blue light is the most influential light on whether or not your child will get a good night's sleep. The sun produces most of the blue light we are exposed to, but LEDs, fluorescent lights, and devices with screens also produce blue light. The light coming from screens, including televisions, computers, tablets, gaming devices, and mobile phones suppresses the production of melatonin and delays your child's ability to fall asleep and stay asleep. Additionally, children may be more susceptible to blue light because they have larger pupils and their sensitivity is higher than adults. Any type of screen or artificial light in the bedroom is a risk factor for poor sleep.

The Outside Environment

The neighborhood you live in can influence how well your child sleeps, too. As mentioned earlier, challenging socio-economic circumstances place children at higher risk for lack of sleep. One study found that children who lived in neighborhoods that had the least health-promoting amenities, like safe areas to play or the presence of sidewalks, had up to 43 percent higher odds of experiencing serious sleep problems.

> **#TruthBomb:** A third of children who report sleep problems in childhood experience sleep difficulties ten years later.

Sleep Disorders

Obstructive sleep apnea (OSA), or the repeated partial or complete blockage of breathing during sleep, is one of the major disruptors of quality sleep in children. About 2–3 percent of children are believed to have this condition. Some of the signs of sleep apnea in kids are snoring, pauses in breathing, mouth breathing, nighttime sweating, and poor growth. Unlike adults with OSA who experience daytime drowsiness, children with OSA tend to exhibit behavior problems. Ironically, many of these behaviors are similar to those seen with ADHD, including poor academic performance, poor attention, learning difficulties, behavior challenges, and hyperactivity. In children, the most common culprit of sleep apnea is enlarged tonsils and adenoids.

Obstructive sleep apnea is increasingly seen in children who are larger in size, especially between the ages of six and nine years, and in adolescence. A bidirectional relationship exists: Children with larger bodies have a higher risk for OSA, and children with diagnosed OSA tend to be larger in size. Currently, the incidence of OSA in larger children is as high as 76 percent even after removing tonsils and adenoids.

Sleep apnea is a concern in children with smaller bodies, too, especially if they have allergies or larger tonsils. Alex was an eleven-year-old

Environmental Contributors to Poor Sleep Hygiene in Children

Poor Sleep Hygiene	Examples
Variable Bedtimes	Nightly bedtime during the week fluctuates; no bedtime on the weekends.
Varied Wake Times	Child allowed to sleep "to the last minute" on school days; sleeps in on the weekends to "catch up."
Stimulating Activities Prior to Bedtime	Roughhousing; running around/ chasing child to the bedroom; jumping on the bed.
Falling Asleep Outside of the Bedroom	Child falls asleep on the couch or parent's bed and is transferred to bed later.
Inconsistent Room Temperature	Bedroom is too hot or too cold.
Noisy Environment	Loud TV; talking within earshot of child's bedroom; neighborhood noises.
Ambient Light	Streetlights; night-lights; computer or TV screen left on.
Caffeine Intake	Caffeinated beverages such as tea, coffee drinks, chocolate, and other caffeine-containing foods consumed within 8 hours of bedtime.

boy with OSA who came to see me because he was extremely picky and smaller. He also had difficulty swallowing due to enlarged tonsils and adenoids, which negatively affected his willingness to eat. Once these were removed, his eating and nutritional status improved tremendously, as did his OSA. A recent study found that smaller kids with OSA had a greater tendency for poor height growth and shorter stature. If you suspect your child is not getting good quality sleep, at any size, speak with your doctor about testing and appropriate treatment.

Caffeine

Caffeine is a psychoactive stimulant. It turns on the brain and makes getting to sleep harder. It's recommended that children younger than twelve years old consume no caffeine, and kids older than twelve do so in limited amounts (85 to 100 milligrams per day, or the equivalent of one 8-ounce cup of coffee or two 12-ounce cans of soda). Yet, 73 percent of children consume caffeine on a given day, according to the CDC, which undoubtedly affects their sleep.

Eating Patterns

Some studies in adults have sought to prove a connection between food and better or poorer sleep quality. For instance, both high carbohydrate and high fat intake are associated with poor sleep. Foods such as milk products, fish, and certain fruits, like tart cherries, which have a high dietary melatonin content, and kiwifruit, which has a high serotonin content, have been shown to promote sleep. Both the Mediterranean diet and the DASH diet, as outlined later in Pillar Six, seem to have a positive influence on sleep in adults, too.

Takeaways:

- Poor sleep hygiene makes it harder for kids to get enough quality sleep.
- Light reinforces sleeping and waking, but too much light at the wrong time may interfere with sleep.
- Obstructive sleep apnea and more body fat may impair sleep and cause disruptions in growth, brain development, mood, and behavior.

Set Up a Good Sleep System

The secret to raising a good sleeper is in establishing sleep hygiene—the routines and rituals that nearly guarantee your child will get a good night's sleep—from an early age. It's time for a sleep revolution! Whether it's adjusting the bedtime routine or tackling light exposure, this next section will help you optimize a sleep system and minimize other factors that can interfere with sleep.

Boost Sleep Hygiene

You'll want to systematize a bedtime routine with consistency across the board—even on weekends—to help your child synchronize their sleep-wake cycle. Calming routines an hour before bedtime can ease your child into sleep, such as a bath or shower or other bathroom activities like brushing teeth, story time, or singing a lullaby before bed. Combine a series of predictable activities during the hour before bedtime to calm your child and encourage sleep. Whatever sequence of events you put in place as part of your child's bedtime routine, the most important part is to keep it predictable and recurrent.

If your toddler gets up and down from bed, don't be too discouraged. Toddlers get FOMO (fear of missing out) and may struggle with separation anxiety, which is totally expected for their age and stage of development. Try to give them more control over the process before bedtime, like choosing their pajamas or a bedtime story to discourage conflict and power struggles. Many toddlers nap twice a day, and preschoolers may nap once a day. As kids get older, however, taking naps late in the day or long naps can throw off their sleep pattern, making it harder to fall asleep at night.

Avoid roughhousing, wrestling, games of chase, or other stimulating activities before bedtime. Kids get revved up and this may delay their ability to fall asleep. For older children who may extend their studies into the night, try to stay consistent with the pre-bedtime routine. Encourage homework and other school-oriented activities outside of the bedroom to maintain a strong association between sleep and your child's bed.

Noise can keep kids from falling asleep and can interrupt their sleep, too. Consider the noise level in your home at night. Turn down televisions, talk quietly, and attempt to reduce noise from outside your home, if possible. Some families who live in noisy areas, like a city, have found a white noise machine helps mask outside noise.

Nighttime Light Management

Believe it or not, you can start to encourage good sleep during the day. Try to get your child in natural sunlight in the morning for about thirty to forty minutes. Sunshine helps synchronize and support your child's natural ability to sleep. Even better? Exercise. It keeps the sleep rhythm in alignment, too. Encourage your child to play outside in the morning to create a doubly effective impact.

Artificial light at night may interfere with falling asleep and staying asleep as it keeps your child's brain turned on. Consider replacing LED or fluorescent lights with red lights, as these don't stimulate wakefulness. Darken the room with light-blocking shades to minimize outside light coming in through the windows.

Keep the bedroom a tech-free zone—no television, electronics, or other screens in bed or in the bedroom. Not only does the light from these electronics stimulate wakefulness, but they're also a potential distraction for your child, tempting them to interact. If, for instance, a computer needs to be in the bedroom, consider changing the settings to dark mode. Blue light–blocking glasses can help if your child has to study at night on a computer or use other devices. Consider employing a technology curfew, ending screen exposure one hour or more before bedtime. You'll learn much more on this topic in Pillar Seven.

Eating and Drinking

Discourage caffeine consumption after noon, as caffeine makes it harder to fall asleep at night. If your child drinks caffeine-containing drinks like tea, soda, or even energy drinks, this behavior may disturb their sleep. Even food can disturb the quality of a good night's sleep. Sugary foods, like desserts, or those made with chocolate or coffee, may spark alertness in your child, making it hard to wind down for bedtime.

Late, heavy meals or snacks can interfere with sleep, also. Of course, a light bedtime snack can be helpful for some children, especially if they are younger or in need of extra nutrition, but try to schedule eating an hour before bedtime.

THE WHOLE-CHILD CHECKUP
Sleep

Let's check in on your child's sleep hygiene and habits. Are you cultivating good sleep hygiene? Use the chart on the next page to identify how you're doing: Learner, Striver, or Thriver.

The Learner: Where Do I Begin?

If your child isn't sleeping as well as you'd like, you're in the right place! First, promote consistent bedtimes and wake times, even on weekends. To get started, estimate the ideal number of hours your child needs to sleep each night, based on their age. Remember, younger children need more than older kids do. You may have to reverse engineer bedtime for the 6- to 12-year-old child, working backward from the wake time needed to make it to school on time. For example, if a seven-year-old needs to be at school by 7:30 a.m., and you calculate a wake time of 6:45 a.m., their bedtime will need to be around 7:30 or 8:00 p.m. to ensure eleven hours of sleep.

Next, develop a bedtime routine for the sixty minutes before lights out. When my kids were really little, we bathed them first and then brushed their teeth and hair. They got into their pajamas (or we helped them), picked out a book, and we all hopped into bed to read. Over time, this morphed into each of them reading to themself with a goodnight visit from us. It's expected that the routine will change over time. The point is to be flexible and use a pre-bedtime routine advantageously—to calm your child so they easily fall asleep when the bedtime hour strikes.

Next, address any interfering lights in the bedroom or outside of it. Whether it's ambient light from the street or from a computer

Sleep: Learner, Striver, or Thriver

	Learner	Striver	Thriver
Sleep Routine	Bedtimes and wake times vary day to day. Caregiver struggles with implementing a nightly routine. Child is rambunctious and resists bedtime and is hard to get up in the morning. Child may need naps; sleeps in on weekends.	Parent engages and disengages with sleep routines and timely bedtimes and wake times. Does have successful, calm bedtime routines, just not consistently. Noise is minimized. Child is tired by the end of the day.	Routine bedtimes and wake times are established. Child is compliant and rarely resists or complains. There is a calm, serene atmosphere around bedtime. Parents and child are easily able to re-establish the sleep routine after summer breaks and vacations. Child is well-rested.
Nighttime Light Management	Child has TV and other screens in the bedroom. May stay up and engage with devices past bedtime. Child has trouble falling asleep.	Parent has removed most of the technology from the bedroom. Other lights may be used to quell fear of the dark. Some delay to sleep occurs.	Child gets morning sunlight and activity. The bedroom is a tech-free zone. Extra light is used minimally. Child falls asleep most nights without difficulty.
Eating and Drinking	Child snacks frequently after dinner and consumes caffeine-containing beverages and foods after lunchtime.	Parent limits access to coffee drinks and other caffeine-based foods and drinks. Eating after dinner is light.	Water is the primary beverage around bedtime. If caffeine-containing foods and/or beverages are offered, they appear early in the day. Snacking after dinner is planned, and employed if needed.

screen, mobile phone, or electronic device, make a plan to minimize it. Will you remove screens and create a tech-free zone? That's a good idea! What about night-lights or streetlights? Consider tucking the night-light under a bed and finding some room-darkening shades. In the mornings, open the shades and let the light in! Last, assess caffeine intake and your child's nighttime eating habits. If they're an obstacle to good sleep, downgrade, eliminate, or alter them.

Any and all of these steps may feel like a huge leap, especially if your child resists and puts up a fuss. It's okay. As with all of the Pillars, you don't have to do it all at once. Pick one thing, focus on it, and move on to the next thing. If these steps aren't working and your child is still struggling to sleep well, you can look for extra help. Talk with your doctor and determine if you need to pursue a sleep study or meet with a sleep specialist or sleep coach.

The Striver: Let's Level Up

Maybe you've got a lot of this figured out. That's great! Leveling up is all about going for the daily habit. If you've got a weekly routine with bedtime going well, apply it to the weekend. Or, if that isn't 100 percent realistic, take the bits and pieces that are working and add them to the weekend routine. For instance, if washing up and reading a book helps your child ease into sleep, then do it on the weekends, too. The most important thing about weekend sleep is that the routine is in place, and the sleep duration is similar to that which occurs during the week. You don't want your child making up sleep with thirteen- or fourteen-hour nights on the weekends, as it may mess up their ability to sleep well during the week.

Maybe you have bedtime established, but wake times are inconsistent. Try to firm them up. If there's too much light in your child's bedroom or they need a night-light, you can ease into darkening the room. If electronics aren't allowed, but some exceptions have crept in, try to get back to a tech-free zone every night. Remember, if you're getting resistance from your child, especially if they're a preteen, have a conversation about all you've learned about sleep in this chapter. Partnering with your older child on the Pillars of Wellness will go a long way toward building shared values and internal motivation.

The Thriver: Keep Up the Good Work

Bravo! Sleep is sneaky in that you may not know the impact of a good night's sleep on your child, but you will know if your child isn't experiencing restorative sleep. If your child appears to be well-rested, alert during the day, productive, and functioning well, they're probably sleeping well. Good work. Keep it up. Sleep is a Pillar of Wellness that will be tested as your child grows. Stay on top of it and keep giving them the gift of this healthy habit.

When you see someone putting on his Big Boots, you can be pretty sure that an Adventure is going to happen.

— A. A. MILNE
(from *Winnie-the-Pooh*)

· ·

PILLAR THREE

· ·

MOVEMENT
As You Like, Every Day

Kids are wired to move. Some seem to be naturally athletic or sporty, and others are not so much. Peter, whom you met in the Introduction, liked to read, play video games, and watch television. When I first started working with him, he was a big-for-his-age boy and his parents wanted him to move more. They understood the benefits: confidence, health, and stress reduction. The challenge was in finding something he enjoyed doing. "Peter would be very happy to come home from school and play video games or read a book," said Ann, his mom. "It's an effort to find something he enjoys, but I know it's important that he's active."

Over the years, Peter tried a number of sports. On the field, he wasn't as fast as the other boys. As a result, he shied away from field sports. He was tall for his age, so basketball was a natural draw. He worked with his basketball coach to hone his shooting skills and became adept at scoring baskets. He played tennis and tried rowing, swimming, and cycling. By the time he was twelve, he'd played a number of team sports and other activities to stay active. He added strength training and tennis. He trained twice a week with his coach in the gym, and played tennis a couple of times a week during the school year and more often in the summer. Peter became stronger, more confident, and enjoyed daily movement.

Although our bodies are meant to move, society emphasizes convenience and attitudes that forgo movement. We take the escalator instead of the stairs. We drive instead of walk. We use washing machines instead of scrub boards. All of these modern conveniences are welcome on many levels, but they've robbed us of the natural, baked-in opportunities for daily movement. As a side dish, we've developed a propensity for sedentary, automated movement. We need to change that—especially for our kids. Movement is a habit that can—and should—start early. It's essential for all children, no matter their size. It helps them grow and develop, prevents chronic diseases, and improves their mental health. It's not always easy to get children to move, but the goal is to help your child enjoy movement and make it part of the daily routine.

WHAT DOES IT MEAN TO BE PHYSICALLY FIT?

Physical fitness is the ability to harness what the body can do physically. It includes:

Cardiorespiratory fitness: The ability of the heart and lungs to deliver oxygen to muscles during exercise at moderate-to-vigorous intensities, and for a period of time.

Musculoskeletal fitness: A measure of muscle strength, endurance, and power to perform work.

Flexibility: The range of motion a group of muscles and joints can experience.

Balance: The ability to maintain equilibrium while moving or not.

Speed: An indicator of how fast your child can move their body.

SCIENCE AND SOCIETY
Why Every Body Should Move

P hysical activity is part of the maintenance routine for a healthy body. Like a car needs to get out on the highway and run its engine, young bodies need to accelerate now and again, too. Activity shouldn't be about changing your child's size. Movement should feel good and be fun—this is the key to building a daily habit. But before we get into how to build this habit, you need to understand the science behind physical activity for children and what it actually does for them.

What Is Movement?

Movement is a term that encompasses physical activity and exercise. According to the World Health Organization (WHO), physical activity is "all movement including during leisure time, for transport to get to and from places, or as part of a person's work." For kids, standing up after sitting in class, taking the stairs to the bathroom, walking to school, or playing on the playground fall under the definition of movement. Exercise, on the other hand, is an intentional physical activity done in an effort to improve health and well-being. This could be joining a gym class, running, swimming, or playing a sport. Exercise involves heavier breathing, a raised heart rate, and sweating.

Any type of movement is beneficial for your child. While there are different degrees of movement throughout the day, they all add up. Sedentary behaviors like sitting on the couch watching TV, or lying around for hours on end, do the opposite. They erode your child's physical health and may add to mental health concerns.

The Benefits of Movement

Physical activity has the power to help your child grow and develop optimally, feel better, prevent the most common chronic disease conditions, and sleep better. Even small amounts of movement can improve health, and the benefits can be seen *immediately* after movement. Physical activity builds muscle and bone strength, improves endurance, and strengthens the heart and lungs. Here's how it can positively affect your child's overall health and well-being:

Heart and Lungs: Physical activity strengthens the heart (a muscle), enabling more blood to pump throughout the body to deliver oxygen to muscles, lungs, and other organs.

Bones and Muscles: Activity helps bones develop, leading to higher bone mass, better bone structure, and more bone strength. Movement also improves muscle function and overall strength in children.

Body Fat: Movement balances energy and encourages healthy amounts of body fat. Children who are larger and who routinely move have better body composition, including lower levels of body fat and abdominal fat.

> **#TruthBomb:**
> Physical activity and exercise are better at maintaining body size than changing it.

Brain Health: Physical activity improves performance on academic achievement tests, executive function skills, processing speed, and memory, not only in the moment of movement but also when daily physical activity is a habit. Exercise and movement can lighten the mood, and even prevent depression by raising dopamine, the feel-good chemical.

Blood Sugar and Fats: Movement improves insulin sensitivity, helping to normalize blood sugar levels and prevent chronic conditions like type 2 diabetes. Regular physical activity also reduces the harmful blood fats (triglycerides) that contribute to heart disease and increases those that are protective.

The Threat of Sedentary Behavior

Sedentary activity is a misnomer. There is no activity in being sedentary. When it comes to kids, being physically inactive means lying down, sitting, or reclining. And yes, a sedentary lifestyle can turn into a habit. While physical activity has many health benefits for your child, being *inactive* has the reverse effect: a higher risk of heart disease, cancer, high blood pressure, type 2 diabetes, extra body fat, and more. "Sitting for a long period of time uses a completely different metabolic pathway and is an independent risk factor for a whole slew of negative health outcomes," says Dr. Rebecca Hasson, associate professor of kinesiology and nutritional sciences at the University of Michigan and director of the Childhood Disparities Research Laboratory. "Even if you've done all this exercise—for two or three hours—if you do a ton of sitting or lethargic sedentary behavior the rest of the day, you are actually counteracting some of those health benefits."

Physical Activity Intensity

Intensity of Activity	Definition	Examples
Sedentary Activity	Awake and sitting, reclining, or lying down	Watching TV, reading a book, playing video games
Light-Intensity Activity	Heart rate isn't elevated, activity can be sustained for at least 60 minutes	Folding clothes, washing dishes, standing in place, painting/arts and crafts, getting dressed
Moderate-Intensity Activity	Heart rate is faster than usual, breathing harder than normal, conversation can be maintained	Walking to school, jumping, bicycling, yoga, gymnastics, slow dancing, shooting a basketball, softball/baseball, social tennis
Vigorous-Intensity Activity	Heart rate is much faster than usual, breathing is much harder than usual, sweating, unable to maintain conversation	Jogging/running, hiking, biking (more than 10 mph), high-impact aerobics, most competitive sports, skiing/snowboarding, roller-skating, steady swimming
Near-Maximal or Maximal Activity	Intense activity that can't be sustained for more than 10 minutes	Sprinting, racing, spurts of intense competitive activity

How Much Do Kids Need to Move?

Younger children tend to play as their primary form of physical activity. It's also natural for them to be intermittently active, doing spurts of activity here and there. As kids get older, their activity patterns change. They participate in extended activities, like playing on a sports team, or participating in gym class. Rather than bursts of activity, school-age children can sustain activity for longer periods. The good news is *any* type of activity, no matter the duration, counts toward achieving the goal of daily movement. Some amount of movement will always be beneficial compared to inactivity.

The health and well-being gains that come from movement increase as the intensity and duration build up. When a car idles, it doesn't burn much fuel. However, when the engine revs and the car moves, the fuel burn is greater. This is true with bodies, too. Even though getting up from the couch is considered physical activity, it is less intense than running across the backyard, which increases the heart rate and engages the muscles. As such, physical activity is broken down by intensity: light intensity, moderate intensity, vigorous intensity, and near maximal activity. These intensities differ based on the rate of energy expenditure (calories burned) compared to sitting at rest. For kids, most health benefits come from moderate-to-vigorous activities.

The intensity of an activity is relative to a child's physical state. A child who isn't used to physical activity may experience walking as a vigorous activity, while a child who is regularly active may experience it as light. Additionally, the intensity can vary. Your child could stroll or walk slowly, they could pick up the pace with purpose, as in walking to school, or they could rush to catch up with friends. The intensity of movement can be all over the place each day, but the more time your child spends moving everyday with a variety of intensities offers the greatest benefits to your child.

> **#TruthBomb:** Children and adults spend more than 7.7 hours per day, or 55 percent of their awake time, being inactive. During the COVID–19 pandemic, children aged five to thirteen years spent about ninety minutes sitting in front of screens for school activities and *over eight hours* of sitting during the day engaging in leisure-related activities like watching TV.

Children aged six years and older should accumulate *three hundred minutes of physical activity per week*. This might be sixty minutes each day for five days per week, or forty to forty-five minutes every day of the week. For younger children, the focus of physical activity should be on play. As kids get older, activities should vary and center on three types of movement: aerobic (heart and lung capacity), muscle building, and bone building.

Goals for Physical Activity

Age	Type of Movement	Examples
3 to 5 Years Old	Play a lot. Play promotes movement and builds brain architecture and resilience. Encourage active play and lots of different activities.	Get outside (backyard, local park, or the driveway). Throwing/catching a ball, riding a tricycle, hopping, playing tag, skipping, jumping, gymnastics/tumbling, swimming, or dancing. These activities offer aerobic, muscle- and bone-strengthening properties.
6 to 13 Years Old (and up to 17 Years)	300 minutes of moderate-to-vigorous physical activity each week, including: **Aerobic activity:** Sweaty, heavy breathing activities; 3+ days per week. **Muscle-strengthening activity:** Strength-building and resistance activities; 3+ days a week. **Bone-strengthening activity:** Impact with the ground or a rapid change of direction; or 3+ days a week.	**Aerobic:** Running, hopping, jumping rope, swimming, dancing, doing martial arts, and riding a bike. Playing a sport. Benefits occur whether activity is brief or extended. **Muscle-strengthening:** Climbing a tree, playing tug of war, lifting weights (with supervision), or using resistance bands. **Bone-strengthening:** Ball games, hopscotch, jumping rope, or running.

Here's where the news about movement gets even better. *A single session* of moderate-to-vigorous activity can lower blood pressure, improve the body's use of insulin, help with better sleep, lower symptoms of anxiety, and improve cognitive function *within the day* that the exercise occurred. When movement occurs every day, the health benefits are magnified. For instance, children with a chronic condition like type 2 diabetes may reduce their long-term risk and improve overall body health and function *within days to weeks* when they participate in regular sessions of moderate-to-vigorous physical activity.

Takeaways:

- Kids need to move their bodies every day.

- Younger children should actively play, and older kids should participate in a combination of enjoyable activities that encourage aerobic, muscle-, and bone-strengthening.

- Any type of movement aids in improving body function, including that of the brain, heart, and lungs, and in regulating blood sugar and body fat.

OBSTACLES AND OBJECTIONS
Why Every Body Isn't Moving

Moving seems like it would be an easy habit to embrace, but it isn't. From time and money constraints to competing desires, setting up this habit for your child can feel like another task on the to-do list or another appointment on the schedule. While there have always been roadblocks to establishing a daily movement habit in children, the COVID-19 pandemic single-handedly made things so much worse. In the face of stay-at-home orders, school closings, working from home, and schooling from home, children and their families struggled to find ways to move regularly. And after years of pandemic disruption, we're all recovering from the toll it's taken on our daily habits, especially around physical activity.

Some of the latest statistics indicate that only 23 percent of eleven-year-olds and 19 percent of thirteen-year-olds achieve the recommended sixty minutes of moderate-to-vigorous activity each day. When I was a kid, my mom sent me outside to play after homework was done. I was encouraged to stay outside until dinner. I roamed the neighborhood on my bike; stopped at the neighborhood empty lot; and played football, kickball, or hide-and-seek. Today's kids, however, are encouraged to stay inside. There's been a shift in values from getting fresh air to getting ahead. Parents, teachers, and the education system value academic achievement over movement. There's also worry about the safety of children. Fear of strangers, injuries, crime, and other dangers have parents keeping their kids indoors. Not to mention that most modern innovations make it convenient and easy to do things without actually having to move. Just think of the automobile, a term that literally suggests we "automate mobility." The computer, smartphone, television, and entertainment devices— all recent innovations—scream *Sit down and engage with me!*, putting movement on the back burner.

The solution for some families is to enroll their kids in structured activities like sports or dance. In fact, the trend of replacing unstructured play with structured activities is happening across the country. But it leaves out kids who lack access to these activities. As a result of these and other obstacles, today's kids get outside less frequently and stay outside for shorter durations. Yet time outdoors has been linked to more physical activity, better physical fitness, and less sedentary behaviors in children between ages three and twelve years.

The Lived Environment

Your lived environment—where you live and your surroundings—may or may not be an obstacle to physical activity. Think about living in the deep woods versus suburbia versus the inner city. These environments make a difference in whether or not movement is, or becomes, a daily habit. In suburban areas, the need for transportation is greater due to large open spaces and a lack of sidewalks. Even inner-city living areas don't necessarily offer more opportunities for movement. Yes, there may be plenty of sidewalks to walk on, but there are different challenges. Dense, crowded living spaces often translate to fewer open green spaces and more considerations for safety.

Where you live offers natural opportunities for movement, or not. "We have effectively engineered out physical activity in our daily lives," says Dr. Hasson. The good news is if you live where there are sidewalks, parks, bike lanes, greenways, playgrounds, fitness facilities, and green spaces, your child may be more inclined to be active, especially if you accompany them and are physically active yourself. The bad news is if you aren't active in this motion-favoring environment, it can have the opposite effect, weakening or eliminating its positive influence.

As you've heard more than once in this book, how you conduct your life translates to how your child conducts theirs. And this proves true when it comes to daily movement. It turns out parenting has a significant impact on whether a child will be active or not. For one, if you're a role model of daily movement, your child is more likely to adopt this habit. And when you support what is needed for physical activity—getting your child out the door, providing access to equipment, and transportation—their moderate-to-vigorous physical activity may *increase* over time, negating the idea that kids become less active as they age. Regular support and the model of your daily habits moves your kid to move.

Schools: A Missed Opportunity

Our society emphasizes achievement and advancement as the keys to success. It leads schools to prescribe lengthy homework assignments and parents to hire tutors and crowd the evenings with other activities in the name of "getting ahead." These values have led to an educational system that fosters physical *inactivity*. Yet, ironically, movement is tied to greater academic performance and better mental health. Doesn't it seem counterproductive to weed it out of schools?

Children should be able to capture some of the minutes they need for moderate-to-vigorous movement at school. But that's not happening. Over the last couple of decades, schools have eliminated opportunities for movement, especially moderate-to-vigorous physical activity. In fact, these opportunities have been steadily declining in schools across the globe by about fifteen minutes per school day.

Additionally, the *actual* physical activity during physical education (PE) classes has declined and children's scores in physical fitness have also plummeted. Funding for physical education programming has dried up, too. "PE has been underfunded and removed from many schools, and recess has been limited," says Dr. Hasson. "There's little time for free play or structured movement for kids at school." This is especially challenging for young bodies that naturally want to move, and even more so for those children who may naturally need more physical stimulation.

THE IMPACT OF THE COVID-19 PANDEMIC

Even though physical activity at school has been dwindling for years, at least older kids walked from classroom to classroom, and younger kids had some time outdoors to play. Not so during the COVID-19 pandemic. Children cut their usual steps from walking around school by 43 percent during the pandemic. Physical activity dropped significantly among children, too, especially middle school youth and teens.

Cardiorespiratory Fitness: A Better Indicator of Health

"I've been fat my whole life," said Nina, an active woman in her mid-forties who golfs, rows, and exercises daily. "Thank goodness I was an active child, running around outside and playing sports. It's allowed me to stay healthy—and it's been a way of life for me." Can children with larger bodies be as active as their peers who are smaller or mid-sized? Size and exercise assumptions aside, children with larger bodies are very capable of moving and can participate in aerobic exercise and weight training. All children benefit from physical activity and should be moving regardless of their size.

Physical activity is an effective tool for improving overall health, as you've learned, but in children with larger bodies, it has been used as a tool for promoting weight loss. The message has always been "move more," with the intention of weight loss. This has caused many unintentional consequences for larger-bodied kids, including shame about their bodies and a lack of motivation to move. A recent study questioned this approach, suggesting that a focus on fitness is a better way. The study argues that cardiorespiratory fitness is a better end goal and indicator of health—a *vital sign* of health—rather than weight or BMI measurements, especially in people with larger bodies. If heart and lung

> **#TruthBomb:** All children can improve their cardiorespiratory fitness and be fit through daily movement, at every size.

function are the *real* indicators of fitness, then *any* individual can be fit, regardless of their size. What a revelation! A focus on fitness also skirts the problematic cycle of dieting and minimizes the threats to mental health and well-being. The American Heart Association (AHA) agrees. Improving cardiorespiratory fitness has better health outcomes for youth.

We should never discourage physical activity based on the size of a child. Aside from the presence of injuries, such as a fracture, ligament tears, or joint problems, all children can move. Even children with chronic health conditions like asthma, epilepsy, or cancer benefit from physical activity. If you have a child with a chronic condition, check in with your doctor, but understand that regular physical activity helps *all* bodies function better.

The Motivation to Move

One complaint I hear from parents is that they can't motivate their children to move . . . or eat healthfully . . . or make the bed. How do you get a child to do anything? Most of us know that threats of punishment or forcing exercise won't work to *really* motivate them long term, but we're not sure how to build motivation that lasts. The key is in understanding motivation. Motivation is the internal desire to do something. It's a powerful ally in developing habits. Yet a lack of motivation can be a barrier to physical activity and any other habit you're trying to cultivate. Before we move into my tips for establishing a habit of daily movement and how to motivate your child in the right ways, let's make sure you understand extrinsic and intrinsic motivation.

Extrinsic motivation is the desire to do something for a reward, or to avoid something, like punishment. For instance, your child may work to get good grades because you'll pay them money for A's and B's, or because they want to avoid punishment (or something unpleasant, like your disappointment). Earning money or avoiding disappointment are external motivators. Another example is providing dessert when your child eats their vegetables or the threat of punishment if they don't eat them. Dessert, or avoiding the loss of story time, are the external rewards that motivate your child to dig into broccoli. While external rewards can elicit behaviors you want to see, they may not result in lasting motivation or good habits. Will your child eat the veggies if you don't offer dessert? Will they work hard for good grades if there's no monetary reward in the end?

Intrinsic motivation, on the other hand, is doing something because it's personally rewarding. A child might work hard to get good grades because they desire a top ranking in their class or enjoy doing well in school. Your child may eat vegetables because they enjoy the taste of them (isn't that the goal?!). Building intrinsic motivation is more likely to be long-lasting. It sustains behaviors in the long run. Obviously, if

WHAT BUILDS INTRINSIC MOTIVATION?

Psychologists highlight three key areas to focus on when building motivation that lasts:

Autonomy is the perception that one controls their own behavior; they have choices, and personal goals are essential for their success. Example: a child can choose [physical activity, snack, timing of chores] based on options that reflect their interests.

Competence is having skills and being able to show them off. It's also the ability to learn new skills while focusing on the growth process rather than the end result. Example: getting better at a sport over time; making one's own snack based on preselected options; trust and respect for doing a good job with chores.

Relatedness refers to the connections one has with others and how it feels to engage in certain behaviors. Example: making friends on a sports team or at an after-school activity encourages attendance.

your child loves a sport or playing outside, it won't be hard to engage them in these physical activities because doing them will be internally rewarding and enjoyable, driving more movement. Ironically, your task isn't in getting your child to move, it's in building and sustaining their intrinsic motivation.

How your child perceives their physical abilities—or what researchers call their *physical self-concept*—also plays a role in their motivation to move. A study of seven- and eight-year-olds looked at whether they needed positive feedback during physical activity to develop a positive self-concept and improve their performance (extrinsic motivation), or whether they needed to *see* themselves as good at physical activity to increase or maintain their motivation (a high physical self-concept). Through a series of questions testing levels of motivation and physical self-concept, paired with a physical performance test, both physical self-concept and intrinsic motivation were associated with better physical activity performance scores, while positive praise was not. Girls and children with larger bodies demonstrated a lower physical self-concept and lower performance scores overall. As young children are at a prime time for developing their physical self-concept and internal desire to be active, efforts to instill regular physical activity need to promote a high physical self-concept and the pleasure of movement, especially in girls and children with larger bodies. These children may also need activity adaptations to reflect their individual capabilities, positive feedback to enhance their physical self-concept, and an emphasis on pleasure in order to have success. Otherwise, their desire and motivation to be active may be stifled.

#TruthBomb: If you use rewards for activities children *already* enjoy, their internal satisfaction may fade. And if you overuse external rewards (or unpleasant consequences), it may negatively affect their motivation.

So, should you nix rewards? No. A reward can help kids get started with new behavior and reinforce it, which can take on intrinsic value over time. Rewards may increase feelings of competence, especially after an accomplishment, and this increases enjoyment. Joy builds intrinsic motivation, which keeps the habit going. For children who aren't necessarily aware that they're building a habit, the focus should be on enjoyment, playfulness, and how it all feels.

The antithesis of building motivation is pushing children to be active in the wrong ways. For instance, forcing a child to exercise can lead them to dread movement. Making a child earn food, like dessert, by exercising a certain amount also backfires. The same goes for shaming a child into exercise, such as stating they need to move more or bulk up due to their size. Shame and stigma will always be demotivators.

Takeaways:

- Where you live and whether you move regularly are strong influences on whether or not your child is physically active.

- Opportunities for movement outside of the home, particularly in schools, have been declining for decades.

- Building internal motivation will keep your child moving, but pushing them to be active by using rewards or punishment can deter their enjoyment and interfere with building a daily habit.

HOW TO STRIVE AND THRIVE
Get All Bodies Moving

Now that you've learned why physical activity is so beneficial to your child, and know the common obstacles that get in the way, let's get to the goods. How do you cultivate a daily habit of movement while building your child's internal motivation to participate? We're going to focus on three areas: preparing your environment, harnessing motivation, and making movement a family affair.

Prep Your Environment for Success

Set up your home, surrounding environments, and daily routines so that it's easier to move. In other words, make movement a no-brainer. Tailor activities to your child's age and build in variety to promote all the benefits we've discussed. Whether you live in an area that is conducive to walking and playing, or you have to make do with indoor pastimes, there are ways to set your child up for success.

Prioritize and schedule daily movement. It pains me to say it, but life is so busy, you need to plan, prioritize, and schedule your child's daily movement. If you don't, it's not likely to happen. "Until there are some larger scale policy changes, families are going to have to take a bit of initiative and schedule it in," advises Dr. Hasson. A plan for movement will help you stay on track and keep your child building this daily habit.

Set up routines that you follow day in and day out. It might be that you walk with your kids to the bus stop or to school. Or, after lunch, everyone goes outside. You could take a daily walk with your little ones after breakfast, or with the whole family after dinner. Encourage your child to go outside after school is done. Or, if you've got a sporty kid, take them to practice and games.

Keep it age-appropriate. Young children enjoy playing. They just need the opportunity to do so. Take them to the park or playground, let them out in the backyard, or block off the driveway so they can ride their trikes or bikes. Even playing inside can work. If your child is playing "house," place some of the "rooms" upstairs or in another part of your home so there's some movement happening. For children, it's important to allow them some freedom, whether it be running around the neighborhood, building a fort in your backyard (or basement), making up dance routines inside, joining friends at the playground, or participating in a neighborhood game of kickball. Just put parameters around safety.

Pay attention to your child's natural interests. I have a picture of my son with a wad of gum in his mouth looking extremely bored out in left field at a baseball game. He was six or seven years old and very uninterested in baseball. It was easy to see. We finished the season and moved on. Pay attention to your child's interests. While you may want them to play soccer, they may be more interested in gymnastics or dance. Observe which interests and activities draw your child in and go from there.

You're not going to get the sport or activity right every time, but you have to start somewhere. Don't get too attached to a specific activity, especially when your child is younger, because kids change. It's more important to build experiences and a variety of skills rather than latch on to one thing. You're on a big adventure when it comes to finding the physical activities your child enjoys.

Embrace free and fee-based activities. I always say free is great. It's free to take a walk, explore your local rivers and trails, play in the park, ride a bike, or follow an exercise video on YouTube. If a fee-based activity is within your budget, there are many options like sports, dance classes, gym memberships, community center programs, and more. Fee-based activities work well for many kids, but remember, most of these don't happen every day, so think about how your child will be active during the off days.

Harness Motivation

The goal here is to tap into internal motivation so your child builds a desire to move and it lasts. Keep these motivation principles in mind as you move through the other habits in this book. Here's how to build your child's motivation to move:

Embrace FEEL. Fun Exercise Enhances Life (FEEL) is an acronym to remind you that building physical activity habits should center on creating *the feeling of fun or playfulness* during any experience. Not only does an experience that's fun turn on internal motivation, it also engages the brain's reward center. And play is intrinsically motivating. To highlight the FEEL factor, your child can self-assess their mood, energy, and joy during physical activity through drawing, journaling, or conversation afterward. For example, have your child draw a picture or write down answers to these questions: *How did your (body, heart, lungs, brain, arms, legs, etc.) feel when you were [physical activity]? How was your energy level (before, during, and after)? What did you enjoy about [physical activity]?*

Foster autonomy, relatedness, and competence. Self-determination theory, or how a person becomes motivated to start new health habits and maintain them over time, relies on autonomy, relatedness, and competence.

When you can, let your child make choices about physical activity. Will they go to the park or the rec center? Will they play soccer this fall or take a martial arts class? The act of choosing taps into your child's autonomy and increases the likelihood that they will enjoy the activity. Of course, expose your child to different activities to learn more about what they enjoy, their emerging interests, or areas of development. Whatever options you present, make sure your child can relate—that there's an interest, a desire, a friend, or another relatable element that will engage them. Last, promote competence— or a sense of mastery—by challenging your child just enough. When things are a bit challenging, motivation is captured, but if it's too hard, motivation may be lost. Focus on the effort, not your child's end results or ultimate performance. When we focus on performance outcomes, such as winning a race, hiking to the top of the mountain, or getting in a certain number of steps, children may become *less* motivated, develop negative attitudes about physical activity, and view their personal abilities pessimistically. Instead, emphasize effort and mastery to build their long-term motivation.

> **#WiseAdvice:**
> Focus on socializing, not specializing. Being social during physical activity builds skills in communication and increases fun and enjoyment. Specializing in a sport may introduce too much pressure and stress, undermining joy. Furthermore, being with friends or family during physical activity is crucial for establishing a habitual and long-lasting internal desire to move.

SHOULD CHILDREN TRACK THEIR PHYSICAL ACTIVITY?

Today there are numerous activity trackers available. Many teens and adults use them to log their steps or track their time exercising. Tracking physical activity may be motivating for some children, but for others it may drive an unhealthy focus on numbers and take the joy out of movement. You know your child best. Focus on the joy of movement and don't connect tracking devices to outcomes, especially a change in body size.

Use empowering words. How you talk about physical activity matters, too. Language may encourage pride and deepen motivation. But perception is everything. Rather than saying "Just do it," reframe it to something more empowering like, "You can do it. You're tough and strong. You've got everything you need to do this." Be careful to avoid stigmatizing remarks about bodies and exercise, as they may undercut motivation and instill shame.

Create Natural Opportunities to Move

Whether you are outside or trapped inside due to the weather, no matter the circumstance:

Get outside more. When it comes to being active, the low-hanging fruit is getting outside. More time outdoors increases the chance your child will get the moderate-to-vigorous activity they need. Don't let the weather dissuade you. Whether it's backyard play, a quick walk to the park, shoveling snow, stacking wood, pulling weeds, going to the local pool, or gardening, being physically active doesn't mean you have to plan an elaborate trip to the park or the mountains. Just get your child out the door. They'll figure out what to do next.

Insert physical activity in unlikely places. When your child is indoors, transform sedentary activities into active ones, such as sitting on a stability ball instead of a chair, standing while playing video games (instead of sitting or lying down), watching television while riding a stationary bike or slowly walking on a treadmill, or using an easel for arts and crafts. You can also build movement into indoor play. For instance, if you have a LEGO builder, encourage your child to use all four corners of the room. Playing "house," creating dramatic plays, or other imaginary scenes with toys can be done in the same way, using the entire room or extending throughout the house. This way, walking, stair-climbing, and general movement are involved. Indoor play doesn't have to be contained in one room. Even cleaning up after playtime is an activity!

Move together! The family that plays together, stays together. As in all health-promoting habits, when your family does it together, it's more likely to become ingrained and habitual. Find new opportunities to be active together. Make tweaks to your daily routines so that you can naturally build more opportunities for movement together.

THE WHOLE-CHILD CHECKUP
Physical Activity

N ow that you know about physical activity, let's see how you're doing, and more important, how your child is doing with daily movement. Are you a Learner, Striver, or Thriver?

The Learner: Where Do I Begin?

The first thing to do is an assessment of your child's physical activity. Jada walks her two elementary kids to school every day and they walk home with friends (fifteen minutes each way). After school, both kids play outside with their neighborhood friends (forty-five minutes). One day a week, each child goes to sports practice (sixty minutes). On weekends, there's a sports game or the family does some sort of outdoor activity, such as a hike, bike ride, or walk in their downtown area (thirty to sixty minutes). Jada's family is active. However, if her kids took the bus, things would look very different. A handle on how much daily movement your child gets plus an understanding of your environmental opportunities are keys to increasing and establishing the movement habit.

If your child isn't moving as much as you'd like, the first thing to tackle is your current home and surrounding environment. What can you optimize? If you have a park, playground, rec center, trailhead, bike trail, or sidewalks, use them. If your outside environment isn't safe for your child or the weather prevents outdoor activity, how can you bring movement opportunities indoors? Take advantage of a piece of exercise equipment, an app, or a video that gets your child moving, or simply set up a play environment in your home that encourages more movement.

Once you've figured out how and where you can build in more activity, get it on the schedule. Write down the times, days, and types of activities for the week, weekends, and different seasons. Look at each day and notice any gaps where daily physical activity is lacking. Consider adding outdoor, indoor, free, and fee-based options.

Physical Activity: Learner, Striver, or Thriver

	Learner	Striver	Thriver
Prepare Your Environment for Success	Child goes out on a nice day but spends quite a bit of time in sedentary activities like watching TV. There's no schedule or plan for physical activity. Family relies mostly on school and playdates.	Parent has signed child up for sports and other activities. Has a good sense of child's interests. Child gets outside some days of the week. Parent is exploring new activities. Starting to set up indoor spaces for more movement.	Child moves daily and is engaged in a variety of activities, hitting the recommended guidelines. Child enjoys play and structured activities. Movement is a natural part of the family routine.
Harness Motivation	Parent decides what activities child participates in. Child may be forced to be active; shamed into moving. Parent is frustrated child isn't more motivated to move.	Parent discusses child's interests with them, coordinating a plan together. Parent understands how to positively motivate the child but may get frustrated when they don't see progress. Parent highlights fun and effort. Child shows internal satisfaction and enjoyment when physically active.	Family empowers child to make decisions about activities, but also has a weekly schedule for a variety of activities. Parent respects and supports their child's daily movement. They embrace FEEL. Child asks to go outside.
Natural Opportunities to Move More	Family doesn't take advantage of the natural environment. Child prefers sedentary activity over physical activity.	Parent is adding natural, easy movement to the day. Parent avoids forcing, negative language, or consequences to motivate movement. Parent is establishing routine activities.	Family has limits on sedentary activity. Family adjusts sedentary activities to be more active. Family empowers child to move the way they like. Daily movement is the norm.

If you're worried about your child's lack of motivation, make sure you're not being too forceful or usurping your child's autonomy. When your child is old enough to have an opinion, sit down and discuss which activities they want to explore. Do everything you can to support your child, and keep noticing their interest level. When your child engages in an activity, speak positively about it, focus on the process, and connect fun and the FEEL factor to optimize motivation. If your child tends to like sedentary activities, like hanging out on screens, start making some adjustments and build more movement into the activity. Always put a positive spin on moving the body no matter your child's age or size.

The Striver: Let's Level Up

You may be feeling pretty good about your child's level of activity. Even if you're in the sweet spot right now, know that this will likely change as your child ages. I encourage you to periodically assess how things are going, especially as the seasons change and your child's interests evolve.

Look for opportunities where your whole family can move together on the weekends. Similar to family meals, moving together offers a time for connection, communication, and new experiences while building self-concept and self-esteem. Can you get a weekly family activity on the calendar? And can you have your child's input on this?

Take advantage of outdoor activities you can only do seasonally, such as skiing, snowboarding, snowshoeing, building a snowman, sledding, or spending the day on the beach. If your child loves to play video games or be on the computer, look for ways to make those activities more "active."

Last, if you see your child happily going out to play, heading to sports practice, or diving into elaborate indoor active play, openly discuss the FEEL factor. No matter the actual feeling—good or not—the conversation alone will plant the seed of internal awareness.

The Thriver: Keep Up the Good Work

Keep going. Enjoyment in moving their body is one of the best habits you can help your child build—it benefits their physical health and their emotional well-being. The biggest thing to remember is to keep all movement fun. Enjoyment will reinforce their motivation and keep your child moving.

Instead of trying to get food into your child,
do your jobs with feeding, then trust him to eat
what and as much as he needs from what you provide.

—ELLYN SATTER

FEEDING

Trust, Love, and Limits

Preparing food, serving it, and cleaning up happens over and over each day. If you have a toddler or preschooler, you're doing it at least five to six times a day (at least that's what is recommended). A middle schooler? Five times, more or less. Not a day goes by without feeding your child. It's a J.O.B. There's nothing in parenting that rivals the energy, consideration, and physical demands of this task. If you have a child who is larger or smaller, or a different eater, such as a picky one or one who is excited by food, feeding them may be harder. "We have tried to nudge and even sometimes force my son to eat new foods, but he ends up gagging, or we sit for an hours-long staring contest," shared Kimberly, mom of a seven-year-old boy. "He's been picky since he was a baby, and now he only eats about twenty foods." The truth is, *any* worry about your child's eating or their body can change how you do your job of feeding.

FEEDING, EATING, AND FOOD

How you feed your child, how your child eats, and the foods that make up your family's diet affect your child's food selections and preferences, their eating habits, and the relationship with food that they develop over time. The difference between feeding, eating, and food can be confusing, so keep the following in mind as you move through the next few Pillars.

Feeding: The interactions and actions you take when offering food, like making what your child wants or restricting certain types of food. Feeding also reflects the attitudes you have about food (good for you, bad for you) and your child's eating performance (too much or too little).

Eating: The process of, and reasons for, consuming food, including the pace of eating, amounts of food consumed, attention to eating, and emotional state.

Food: The substances consumed, which provide nourishment and enjoyment.

In a TEDx talk I gave in 2017, I described the struggle to feed my first child. Once she started solids in the middle of her first year, the interaction between us became stressful. There was a lot of push-pull around food. I urged her to take more bites of food, or I'd remind her to eat. She was disinterested and cut the meal short. We did this dance a couple of times a day. Eventually, she wasn't eating well enough to grow. By the time she was a year and a half, she was also anemic. I share this story often (for more details, you can watch the TEDx talk or read *Fearless Feeding*) to point out that feeding kids can be as powerful to their health and well-being as the food they eat. Even as a health-care professional with deep education and experience in the field of pediatric nutrition, I struggled. While knowledge may not prevent the challenges of feeding your child, it will make you more aware of *why* you or your child are struggling and *how* to overcome it. And this awareness is the heart and soul of this chapter.

Here, you'll learn about feeding, the Pillar of Wellness that encompasses the multiple, daily interactions you have with your child around food. The act of feeding—or providing, navigating, and negotiating food with your child—is a powerful facilitator to their budding relationship with food. What is the relationship with food? It's how your child feels about food and eating it, and it plays a role in your child's body image, self-esteem, and physical health.

SCIENCE AND SOCIETY
The Relationship with Food Starts Here

You prepare food, and you want your child to eat it. But the question *How do I get my kid to eat?* is one with which many parents struggle. News flash! You can't get kids to eat. In fact, the more you *try* to get your child to eat, the worse their eating may get. That's because many of the tactics we use backfire. But we can't help ourselves. Parent feeding comes with its own baggage. If you were fed with certain attitudes and beliefs like "eat everything on your plate before you get dessert," then you may have the tendency to impart these same rules to your child. This is called *intergenerational feeding*, or the passing on of feeding practices to future generations.

Feeding began the day your child was born. You watched for signs of your baby's hunger and you responded with the breast or bottle. When your baby pulled away, you stopped feeding. This is called responsive feeding, and it starts the continuum of feeding, supporting your child's internal capability to regulate their appetite and eating. The opposite is nonresponsive feeding. When a toddler shows signs of fullness, instead of stopping a meal, a caregiver may encourage eating until the meal is finished. Overriding fullness cues by feeding more, or cutting a meal short when a child is not yet satisfied, teaches children to rely on external cues for eating, which can contribute to overeating and loss of appetite regulation. All feeding is responsive, or not. Let's explore how your feeding style and daily interactions help or hinder your child's developing relationship with food.

Your Feeding Style

The research on feeding styles has evolved over the years. Currently there are three main feeding styles of focus: controlling, indulgent, and diplomatic. Caregivers can demonstrate each of these feeding styles every day; however, the tendency is to follow one primary approach. Often, it's the one with which you grew up.

Controlling Feeding Style

I was raised with a controlling feeding style—the "clean your plate" rule was alive and well in my family. Likely ingrained from my parents' own childhoods, as it was for many parents who raised kids in the '70s, the feast or famine mentality came from the ghosts of World War II. This philosophy still exists today and shows up at American tables. Whether you have the privilege of purchasing food from Whole Foods or experience food insecurity, the notion of "eat now because we're not sure if we'll have enough tomorrow" or "eat everything and don't waste food" can play out in everyday feeding.

The controlling feeding style is a top-down, parent-centered way of feeding. Parents make the rules about eating and food and may have low sensitivity to a child's food preferences and appetite. Examples of this include plating a child's meal and expecting them to eat all of it, having a child sit at the table until they finish their meal or eat a particular food, and making dessert unavailable or contingent on eating vegetables (or another food). It doesn't matter whether a child likes the food or is satisfied or full; the child is expected to eat a prescribed amount of food, or type of food, to meet the caregiver's criteria of "good enough."

If you have a child with a larger body, studies suggest you'll be more likely to use the controlling feeding style. Additionally, if *you* have a larger body, you may have the tendency to be controlling to prevent your child from having one. This plays out mainly through what is called *food restriction*, a feeding practice that is linked with a controlling

> **#WiseAdvice:** You can't be both controlling and trusting—they are opposites. Trust your child has the capability to choose and eat food in the right amounts for them. This is the most efficient road to a healthy relationship with food. Being too controlling increases the risk of an unhealthy relationship with food.

feeding style. Limiting food portions or types of food allowed, such as forbidding sugary foods or sweet treats in the home; rationing portions of food, particularly sugary foods; or having a "clean" home, or one with no "junk" foods, are nods to food restriction. We'll cover the downsides of food restriction in the next section.

The controlling feeding style is also prevalent among parents who have children with smaller bodies and plays out as pressure to eat. Nagging, insisting, or suggesting your child take another bite; try or taste this or that food; and giving ultimatums on what and how much needs to be eaten at meals are examples. All parents of children of varying sizes worry about their child's eating, but parents of children who are smaller try harder to get their child to eat, and are more likely to use a controlling feeding style.

HELICOPTER FEEDING

Overprotective feeding, or being a "helicopter parent" at the table, is an emerging feeding style. It's characterized by good things like monitoring food intake, role modeling, and promoting nutritious foods in the home, but it also showcases higher use of pressure to eat and overinvolvement in a child's eating.

Unfortunately, the controlling feeding style significantly interferes with a child's ability to know when to start and stop eating and may contribute to overeating or undereating. For example, in some kids, controlling feeding translates to eating more than their appetite calls for; while in others, it leads to a standoff at the table, poor eating, and a perpetual dislike of food. "When I was a kid, I spent many evenings at the table alone, staring at a portion of green beans on my plate," said Margot. "I wasn't dismissed until I ate them, and to this day, I still dislike green beans." Any means of pressuring your child to eat or controlling their eating can be counterproductive and have long-lasting effects on their relationship with food. Even praise for eating may be interpreted as pressure to eat, dissuading a child from doing so.

Indulgent Feeding Style

Opposing the controlling feeding style is the indulgent feeding style, a child-centered approach characterized by a heightened sensitivity to a child's food preferences, food requests, and a lack of structure with meals and snacks. When describing this feeding style, I often call this the "Yes" feeding approach. The parent wants to say no or set limits, but takes the path of least resistance. For example, Mia's three kids wear her down nearly every day, with their "I'm hungry!" wails, scavenging in the kitchen for food, and refusal to eat at mealtime. She finds herself saying yes, just to avoid the fallout. "Food in my house is pure chaos," said Mia. "My kids are always eating, and I'm exhausted by all the cooking I do just to keep everyone happy."

The indulgent style of feeding is characterized by a loose structure around food and fewer demands on the child. Meals and snacks may not have a regular schedule, access to food is easy, and the parent is more perceptive to their child's appetite and food preferences. If Laura's boys asked to bake cookies or wanted a snack, she said yes. She didn't want them to go hungry or miss out on a "food experience," even though they might not really be hungry. Kids who are raised with the indulgent feeding style have a hard time self-regulating their eating, especially sweets. As such, some children may overeat them.

When you hear about these feeding styles, you may be thinking, *I was fed like this, and I survived.* But at what cost? How do the ghosts of your past food and eating experiences influence your attitudes and actions today? Many of us look back and even chuckle at memories of food and eating. I do when I think of my sister shoving green peas and other vegetables she didn't like down the side of the radiator at dinnertime or adding half a bottle of ketchup to her bean soup. But there are also sad stories and outcomes. Adults with such negative experiences that they vow to never eat certain foods again. Adults who still struggle with eating or negative emotions about food as a result of their childhood experiences. Or those who went down the path of disordered eating or who have health problems. Many parents vow they'll never do to their children what was done to them with food. The good news is there's a better way.

Diplomatic Feeding Style

What if you could feed your child with love while also establishing thoughtful limits that support their healthy relationship with food, physical health, and emotional well-being? I'm here to tell you, yes you can. The diplomatic feeding style gives you this foundation, by emphasizing structure, boundaries, autonomy, trust, and responsiveness. As the name suggests, diplomatic feeding brings "love and limits" to the table.

#WiseAdvice: You have the ability to reparent your food history and repair your childhood feeding experiences by feeding your own child in positive ways.

A diplomatic feeding style is sensitive to a child's appetite and food preferences (this is the love part), yet implements a strategy for feeding that incorporates structure and boundaries (this is the limits part). Let's break this down. Structure is the routine you set around meals and snacks. The opportunities to eat happen with a routine, or schedule, including times for meals and snacks, and spacing between them that's appropriate for a child's age. For example, toddlers and preschoolers have smaller tummies so they need to eat more frequently. Elementary- and middle-school kids have slightly bigger tummies, allowing them to go longer between eating sessions. Setting a routine eating schedule supports a child's appetite regulation because it coincides with their natural digestion and appetite rhythm. More on this in the next Pillar.

The structure also identifies a usual location for meals and snacks, such as the kitchen table or island. Together, the schedule and location build predictability. Think about toddlers and preschoolers going to school. They have a morning routine. They hang up their coats, take off their shoes, and sit in a circle. This predictable routine builds trust and security. They know what to expect and what to do. A routine with eating does the same, creating predictability and providing you a framework with which to feed each day. Of course, you don't need to be strict with mealtimes or the location (nor should you be because I also want you to emulate flexibility). But stick with the routine as much as possible—especially in the early years—to help your child build good eating habits and awareness of their appetite cues.

Boundaries are the second piece to diplomatic feeding. What are boundaries? In short, they're the "no's," or limits on food and eating that support the structure and routines in the home. Ayla, like many moms, felt bad about refusing her child food. "Even though my daughter couldn't possibly be starving because she just ate, I have a hard time saying 'no' to her when she starts to whine," said Ayla. "I feel so mean. What's the big deal anyway?"

As parents, we all have to say "no" to our kids. *No, you can't skip school today. No, you can't ride your bike unless you wear a helmet. No, you can't call your brother names. No, you can't stay up past midnight.* The "noes" feel endless at times. Saying "yes" to food can feel like an easy win. But is it? I've watched kids who hear too many "yeses" rule the roost when it comes to food, having free rein in the kitchen, taking charge of the grocery list, and eating whatever and whenever they want. Although some may argue that this promotes "intuitive eating," my experience is that some kids, especially those with emerging or lower executive functioning skills and higher motivation to eat, may develop problematic eating habits when boundaries are loose or nonexistent. A lack of boundaries may be a serious barrier to cultivating healthful eating behaviors. *That's the big deal.*

Diplomatic feeding is the gold standard of feeding. This is *how* you should feed your child and *how* you want to set up your feeding strategy at home. Why? Because children who are raised this way have better regulation of their eating, have a greater tendency to consume nutritious foods, are more active, have a good relationship with food, and live in a well-functioning body, at every size.

Responsive Food Parenting: Putting It All Together

Food parenting is how you parent around food, but rather than just focusing on your attitude and actions in the kitchen and at the table, it also includes monitoring, modeling, and education. Monitoring your child's eating means understanding what your child is eating (and not eating) throughout the day so you can make adjustments to the menu and get closer to a nutritious eating pattern. For example, if your child eats a birthday cupcake at school, then goes to sports practice and has cookies and a juice drink for a snack, you may choose to skip the dessert you had planned and save it for another night based on this information. This is monitoring at its best, allowing you to take in information about your child's eating and make adjustments to your menu in real time. Monitoring is not to be confused with controlling your child's eating. Rather, it's an awareness of the ebb and flow of eating and the variety of foods that fill your child's day. Role modeling and educating your child about food is part of the gig, too.

Takeaways:

- Feeding styles can encourage (or discourage) children to self-regulate their appetite and eating.

- Feeding styles may set kids up to eat based on external factors or internal cues and can influence the food relationship for better or worse.

- The most productive feeding style is the diplomatic (love with limits) feeding style, which includes mealtime schedules and routines, and boundaries to help kids stay in tune with their appetite and eat with regularity (not too much, not too little).

OBSTACLES AND OBJECTIONS
Counterproductive Feeding

Counterproductive feeding interferes with your child's appetite regulation and eating habits and gets in the way of positive, productive feeding. Of course, busy schedules, a chaotic home, and other socio-economic factors may intrude, but here I'll focus on things that make you more vulnerable to counterproductive feeding.

Parental Factors That Affect Feeding

"I've struggled my whole life with eating, bingeing on sweets and chips, then dieting to get the weight off," said Erica, mom to a ten-year-old girl. "I don't want to pass on these issues to my kid." Erica's desire to protect her child from her own food issues is strong. She's not alone. I've heard this desire before, too many times to count. But before a parent can avoid passing down their baggage to their child, they have to understand it and come to terms with it. Acknowledging your feeding history is a good first step. What was it like to be at the dinner table with your family? Warm, comforting, and accepting? A place you looked forward to being? Or was it a place where you were confronted, uncomfortable, or teased? If you have good memories of feeding, harness the good stuff and use it with your own family. If you have negative memories or emotions, sort through them so you can avoid carrying them forward.

Parent Body Struggles and Feeding

If you struggle with your size, you may be afraid you'll pass your eating habits or health conditions to your child. This fear and how you feel about your body can alter how you feed your child. For instance, you may disengage from feeding because it's too much of a struggle for you personally. Or you may try to control or restrict food (controlling), or be lax (indulgent).

If you have a history of an eating disorder, studies suggest you may have more difficulty feeding your child, manifesting as slower feeding, smaller portions, or a lack of routine with meals and snacks. Furthermore, you may be more inclined to choose "healthy food" or a vegetarian-style eating pattern, restrict amounts or types of food (e.g., sweets), show negative emotions about food, intrude in your child's eating, and have higher concerns about their body size and growth. Parents with past eating disorders may also rate their children as having a difficult temperament and more tantrums, and perceive them to be less happy and active. But there's an upside, too. "When people who have a history of eating disorders become parents, they become really skilled at identifying symptoms of disordered eating and eating disorders early," says Dr. Kendrin Sonneville. "It's a strength they have."

Parent Emotional Health and Feeding

Your emotional well-being may affect your ability to feed well, too. Studies have shown that mothers (and I suspect fathers and other caregivers, too) who have anxiety, depression, or other mental health symptoms may feed in nonresponsive ways. For example, they may be more likely to feed with controlling feeding practices such as food restriction and using food as a reward. Or they may not model healthful eating, or give their children more control over food.

Getting Kids to Eat (Or Not)

When parents use counterproductive feeding, they may interfere with their child's ability to regulate their eating. So what is poor self-regulation? It's an inability to recognize the internal sensations and connection to appetite. For example, let's look at Mia's three kids who were "always hungry." When kids are always hungry, they're either not eating enough food, eating foods that don't contribute to satiety or fullness, or they're simply out of touch with their sense of hunger. When kids graze, snack, or eat frequently, it's common to never feel full *and* never feel hungry. Your child's tummy is near empty when appetite hormones signal hunger. If their tummy is never empty, they never feel true hunger. As such, they can become out of sync with their appetite cues. Certain feeding tactics reduce appetite awareness and interfere with self-regulation.

Food Rewards and Food Restriction

Six-year-old Kelsey loves sweets. Her mother, Marina, is afraid she's obsessed with them. "I'm guilty of bribing my daughter with dessert. It's the only way I can get her to eat vegetables," said Marina. "Lately, though, I've noticed she asks for sweets all the time. She seems very focused on them." It's not uncommon for parents and caregivers to use food rewards to get their kids to eat. And they keep using this strategy because it works! At least in the short term.

Food rewards are generally sweets and treats that are manipulated to get kids to eat other foods or a predetermined amount of food. Kids see food rewards frequently. In schools, they're used to get kids to behave, or are offered in response to achievement. In health-care offices, they may be used to reward good behavior. Long term, food rewards end up changing a child's *perception* of food, setting up a hierarchy where the "reward" food (usually sweets and treats) is valued more than the food a child is being encouraged to eat (often vegetables, meat, or other "healthy" food). In the case of Marina's daughter, Kelsey had learned that sweets were second to none and they became highly desirable. The fact that sweets are tasty and a quick source of "feel good" energy cemented the draw to them. It was plausible that Kelsey would become preoccupied with them.

Not only do food rewards change the way kids view food, but they can also change the quality of the diet and the relationship with food. Furthermore, children may eat despite not being hungry. Although it's not a crime to incentivize your child to eat or reward them for good behavior with a treat, if this is one of your main feeding strategies, it can have some undesirable long-term implications.

The other end of the feeding practice spectrum is food restriction, or making food "forbidden" and creating a sense of scarcity. Typically, foods that are restricted or tightly controlled are sweets and treats. Tightly controlling portion sizes or refusing second helpings may be considered food restriction, too. Making certain foods off-limits may make your child feel anxious and preoccupied about getting them. As a result, some kids adopt food-seeking behaviors, like hoarding food or sneak-eating. When these scarce foods become available, children may overeat them. Intuitively, this is easy to understand. When you go on a diet and all your favorite foods are off-limits, you miss them and think about them. When the diet is over, you may overreact, seeking those forbidden foods, losing control of eating them, and eating too much. These tendencies play out in children, too. The truth is, we all become a little frantic and obsessed with what we cannot have. Especially food.

#WiseAdvice: The temptation to get children with smaller bodies to eat is strong. Watch out for food rewards! Yes, they may work at the moment, but long term, they can crowd out important nutrients, decrease the quality of your child's diet, and set them up for a food fixation, causing more problems with eating habits and health down the road.

Pressure to Eat and Punishment

Nagging a child to eat can be a turnoff. I'd say this is true for most kids, but that depends on their temperament of course. Some kids will obediently follow their parent's requests and eat more, well past their appetite. Other kids will dig in their heels and refuse to eat. Pressure to eat is a slippery slope. On the one hand, you run the risk of teaching your child to overeat by pressuring them to eat more. On the other, you risk disinterest or disgust, and early fullness if your child is smaller or a picky eater. For all children, but especially those at either end of the size spectrum, pressure to eat is associated with poor eating regulation. You could say it's a double-edged sword.

> **#WiseAdvice:** If you've got a child with a larger body, watch out for food restriction. Making food scarce in the hopes of changing the way or how much your child eats can backfire, leading to more food-seeking behavior, eating more, and a distorted relationship with food.

Punishment for eating too much or not enough, such as taking away privileges like toys or TV time, or other disciplinary actions, can have disturbing lifelong implications for children. When Carla shared that her husband yelled at their preschooler for refusing to eat her dinner, I winced. It's not criminal to not eat. In fact, children have the right to refuse food. By allowing them this right, we send the message that we respect their autonomy, bodies, and ability to manage their eating. Punishment doesn't improve eating behaviors, nor does it help a child develop a positive outlook on food and eating. Let's not entangle eating performance and discipline. It drums up all kinds of worthiness, self-esteem, and body challenges, not to mention food issues.

Catering and Chaotic Meals

Kelly was exhausted and tired of making three or four different meals for her family each night. She felt trapped. If she didn't cater to their preferences, they would complain, refuse to eat, and be boorish at the table. "I know I did this to myself," she said. "But I thought it was my job to make sure they ate a decent dinner. Isn't it better they eat *something*, rather than nothing?" If your child is smaller or a picky eater, the inclination to short-order cook to get them to eat *something* is higher. Catering (aka short-order cooking) is defined as making different meals or snacks per a child's request. Although this feeding practice may make you feel like a good mom or dad, if you do it too much, and your child expects it, you may be contributing to more problems. Kids who get a separate or alternate meal, or who take a primary role in deciding what they're eating, may be more likely to have a nutrient deficiency. Additionally, kids who are catered to are less likely to try new foods. This puts parents in a real pickle. Don't worry, there's a way out of this bind. Keep reading!

Ever feel mealtime is a stress bomb waiting to explode? Your child can feel stressed at the table, too. Chaos at the table, including unpredictable meal schedules, children who get up and down from the table, and an environment filled with tension, breeds stress and a negative vibe. Mealtime chaos may lead to eating chaos, making it hard for children to tune in to their appetite and hard for you to enjoy meals. In the end, family meals may become a negative event in which nobody wants to participate. Or worse, one everybody dreads.

Feeding is a dynamic *relationship* between you and your child. What your child does with eating affects how you feed them. And what you do with feeding affects how they eat. Interestingly, parents tend to react to their child's eating more than the child reacts to feeding. If you see yourself in some of these counterproductive feeding practices, the good news is you can avoid negative outcomes. Being aware of your feeding tendencies and how they play out offers you an opportunity to change things, especially if you're struggling in this area. Of course, positive feeding is the way to go. So, let me show you how to do this!

Takeaways:

- Getting kids to eat (or not eat) often engages short-term feeding practices like food restriction, rewards, pressure to eat, and short-order cooking, which can have long-term, negative repercussions.

- A parent's childhood history, feelings about or struggles with their body, and emotional health may alter their feeding approach.

- When children have smaller or larger bodies, counterproductive feeding is more likely to occur.

HOW TO STRIVE AND THRIVE
Positive Approaches to Feeding

A diplomatic feeding style is the key to raising a child who eats well and self-regulates their eating. Here, we'll explore how to set up a structure, use limits to support the structure, and build autonomy and cooperation by involving your child.

The Feeding Strategy: Structure and Boundaries

Structure and boundaries are the foundations of good food parenting. Everything else builds from there. Setting up a structure with meals and snacks is pretty easy, and once implemented, quite powerful for everyone. First, set your times for meals and snacks. This will be dependent on your child's age. The following table gives you an age-related target for the schedule, but this can be modified based on your family's demands and obligations. The goal is to stay on schedule, or as close to it as possible, each day so it's routine and habitual.

Sample Eating Schedules for Kids

Age	Eat Every . . .	Example
Preschoolers (3–5 years) (3 meals + 3 snacks)	2½–3 hours	7:00 a.m. breakfast 10:00 a.m. snack 12:30 p.m. lunch 3:00 p.m. snack 5:30 p.m. dinner 8:00 p.m. snack
Children (6–9 years) (3 meals + 2 snacks)	3–4 hours	7:00 a.m. breakfast 10:00 a.m. snack 12:30 p.m. lunch 3:30 p.m. snack 6:30 p.m. dinner
Preteens (10–13 years) (3 meals + 1–2 snacks)	3–5 hours	7:00 a.m. breakfast 10:30 a.m. snack 1:00 p.m. lunch 3:30 p.m. snack 7:00 p.m. dinner

Next, pick your "usual" location for meals and snacks. Again, eat in this location most of the time so it's predictable. Many families choose to eat in the kitchen, dining room, or a common-use area. When your child understands that meals and snacks happen at predictable times during the day and in a certain location, it takes the question mark away, allowing your child to feel secure. In the big scheme, repeating this mealtime routine day in and day out creates a habit that can lead to better appetite regulation.

Then, think about food and kitchen boundaries. These are the limits that let you say "not now" rather than "no." They also reinforce your meal and snack routine. For example, when your child asks for a snack an hour after lunch, you can say "It's not snack time yet. Let's go outside." Boundaries reinforce the eating schedule, helping your child tune in to appetite cues. But what if your child is *really* hungry? If they didn't eat enough at mealtime or are in a growth spurt, and your intuition tells you they need more food, by all means, give it to them. Offer a piece of fruit or another filling food, have them sit down and eat, then get back to the food routine. The point isn't to be rigid about the routine, or too flexible. Rather, use your leadership, be aware of your child's ups and downs with eating, keenly listen to your child, and make feeding decisions that are useful for the long run.

Choice, Involvement, and Education

Cultivate autonomy by giving your child choices and letting them make decisions. When it comes to food, for instance, keep the choices reasonable, in the same food category, and age-appropriate. For example, offer two choices, like an apple or banana for the preschooler and young child, and three options for the elementary-school-age child and preteen, such as toast, an English muffin, or a bagel. Of course, offer options that are practical for you and available—this is the reasonable part. When kids get to choose, they are more engaged and likely to eat what they've chosen.

Involve your child with food and create opportunities to learn. In a home, there's a natural environment that leads to food education. Take advantage of this! Preparing food, like washing, chopping, peeling, slicing, stirring, and tearing, are all things your child can do (age-appropriately). By doing, they are learning in a natural, hands-on

Food and Eating Boundaries

What You Can Say	The Message It Delivers	How It Helps
"The kitchen is closed right now. It'll be open for [snack, lunch, dinner] at [X] time."	You can't eat right now, but there's a meal or snack in your future.	Maintains the integrity of your routine and encourages appetite awareness.
"In our house, we ask before we help ourselves."	The adult is in charge of food and the kitchen.	Maintains the parent and child roles.
"That's not on the menu today, but we can have that soon [tomorrow, next week, at Grandma's house]."	You can't have what you want to eat right now, but you can have it at a future date.	Sets a limit now but predicts future eating.
"Food stays in the kitchen. Let's sit down and enjoy that snack."	Eating occurs in certain places.	Maintains the routine and the ability to monitor eating.
"You don't have to eat, but I expect you to join family mealtime."	I respect you, but there are expectations to meet.	Allows children to make decisions and learn from them.
"No phones at the table."	This is a distraction-free zone.	Helps your child mindfully focus on food and eating.
"Don't yuck my yum. Use your manners."	We all need to be respectful of food and others at the table.	Sets parameters for acceptable behavior at the table.

way. Responsibilities like household or kitchen chores help your child be more independent and autonomous, which feeds their self-esteem. When kids cook, teach them to clean up. If your child is helping with meal planning, take them to the store to shop for food items. Always try to keep food and food experiences adventurous and fun, but don't forget to convey the responsibility associated with executing meal-times, too.

Serving Family Meals: Plated versus Self-Service

Danielle makes a home-cooked meal most nights of the week. Of the three kids in her family, one child is more choosy than the rest. Danielle plates food and puts it on the table for each family member. "I hate this!" says Charlie, the finicky seven-year-old. From that point on, the atmosphere deteriorates. Dad gets upset at Charlie: "Your mom has worked hard on this meal and you should be grateful and eat it." Seth, the twelve-year-old, complains that Charlie does this every night: "You're a baby! Grow up and eat." Danielle feels badly because the only thing that makes Charlie happy is plain pasta and chicken nuggets. She wonders if Charlie will ever eat more than this, and more important, how she can reverse this devolving family mealtime. "I've tried everything I can think of to make a meal that everyone will eat," says Danielle. "But Charlie is my biggest challenge. I have to make something separate for him."

Parents and caregivers make meals, put them on the table, and their kids respond in a variety of ways. Some happily eat. Other kids whine and complain, refuse to eat, ask for something different, act out, pick at their food, make faces and verbalizations of disgust, and get up and down from the table (avoidance behavior). The reasons for these behaviors are many, such as picky eating, wanting control, or simply pushing the limits to see how far they can go. If your child "whines and dines," you may want to take a different approach to how you serve family meals. Rather than plating the meal as Danielle does, try a self-serve approach. Self-serve meals engage your child's ability to make decisions for themselves and self-govern their behavior. Hello, cooperation! Your child decides what and how much food will go on their plate (from what you've served), which may lead to better eating and greater satisfaction. Also, your child gets exposed to all the mealtime foods. Even if they don't eat them, they see food variety and experience food characteristics, like color and texture.

Here are three different ways you can implement self-service meals:

The Classic Family-Style Table

Imagine a table with platters and bowls of food centered on the table: burgers on a platter, home fries in a bowl, a bowl of salad, a basket of clementines, and a pitcher of milk—a well-balanced, nutritious meal. Instead of putting these foods on a plate, the classic family-style meal encourages family members to pass the food around and take what and how much they want to eat.

Caveats: Toddlers and preschoolers may need help with passing food. An adult can hold the platters and bowls so they can put food on their plate. When planning the meal items be considerate. Take care to include one or two "safe" foods—ones that even the choosiest child will eat, such as milk, bread, or fruit. Note, this doesn't need to be a favorite food, just something your child is familiar with and is inclined to eat.

I'M AFRAID MY CHILD WILL OVEREAT OR NOT EAT AT ALL

If allowing your child to serve themself at mealtimes drums up fears of out-of-control eating or sitting at the table with an empty plate, you're not alone. It's the main argument that prevents parents from giving their child more autonomy at mealtimes. In my experience, when children are allowed to choose what goes on their plate, they are more receptive and excited about mealtime. Kids who have experienced some of the counterproductive feeding tactics described earlier may be exuberant initially and perhaps load up their plates. Others who have been nagged or manipulated to eat may not trust they are free of conditions around food and eating. Kids may need some time to settle in to this new approach to mealtimes.

Self-service meals can help heal any missteps or wounds caused by negative feeding approaches, repairing trust and opening a door to food enjoyment and exploration. Remember, you are in charge of what is served for mealtimes. If you embrace positive feeding, you'll want to let your child be in charge of what goes on their plate and in their body.

Buffet-Style or Smorgasbord

Ever take your child to a party with a spread of food laid out buffet-style? Or go through the smorgasbord at a restaurant? If your child eats well when in this food environment, it's probably because they are in charge of their choices. Kids get to pick and choose what and how much they want to eat, optimizing their autonomy. You can do this at home by laying meal items on an island or kitchen counter "buffet-style," letting your child go through the line and pick their meal or snack.

Caveats: This is a good option for school-age children who can balance standing, holding a plate, and serving themselves. Of course, assist the younger child who needs help and let them tell you what they want on their plate.

DIY and Deconstructed Meals

The Do-It-Yourself (DIY) movement can be applied to mealtime, too. The more we let children do for themselves, particularly with food, the more they learn about it, cooperate with food routines, and gain confidence and autonomy. You can start with small snacks and move to a weekly meal. When my kids were school-age, I dribbled in an occasional YOYO (You're On Your Own) night, which meant they were free to choose what they wanted for dinner from the items I had available and make it for themselves. Sometimes this was reheating leftovers, making a sandwich or bowl of cereal with toast, or coordinating with another sibling to make something simple, like macaroni and cheese. It gave me a night off, but more important, allowed my kids to be independent, which, as you've learned, has far-reaching benefits.

Deconstructed meals are another way to encourage self-service at mealtime. In this approach, you deconstruct or break down the entrée into its parts. For example, tacos can be deconstructed into taco shells, meat, cheese, and other toppings like lettuce, tomatoes, and guacamole. Your child can assemble the taco in any manner. For instance, they may assemble a traditional taco with all the components, a plate with meat and cheese and the taco shell on the side, or a plate with cheese and a taco shell on the side. The end product is completely your child's creation and preference. Of course, you'll have side dishes to round out the entrée, too. Again, when your child can pick and choose what and how things are arranged on the plate, they'll be more likely to eat it. And you'll be fascinated by what they come up with!

Service with a Smile

Positive, pleasant family meals hinge on a positive, pleasant parent or caregiver. Do your best to cultivate and preserve an atmosphere of acceptance, engagement, and loving connection so your child is happy to come to the table. Remember, although the menu is important to physical health, the vibe and interactions at the table influence your child's emotional development and well-being. Smile and laugh more. Critique and complain less. Your attitudes and actions matter!

THE WHOLE-CHILD CHECKUP
Feeding

N ow that you've learned about feeding your child, let's check in on where you're at. Wherever you find yourself, knowing more means doing better. Let's help you take the next step as a: Learner, Striver, or Thriver.

The Learner: Where Do I Begin?

Let's get you on a schedule with meals and snacks first. Do this based on your family's schedule—when adults are home, and your child's scheduling commitments cooperate. Next, figure out snacks. You want the same level of structure (timely intervals and regular location) applied here, too. Then, simply follow the schedule. If your child is not used to having meals and snacks on a schedule, write it down and post it somewhere in the kitchen, like on a blackboard or dry-erase board, so it's obvious and they can refer to it if needed.

Next, work on your kitchen boundaries. You may get some pushback from your child, especially if they're older. Although it may not feel entirely comfortable at first, I want you to solidify your leadership, structure, and routines with food. Boundaries will help you do this. Let's play out the snacking scenario, as it's where many parents get hung up:

Feeding: Learner, Striver, or Thriver

	Learner	Striver	Thriver
Eating Routines	Meals and snacks are not routine. Timing, as well as the location for meals and snacks, is variable. Parent struggles with planning ahead, shopping, and cooking.	Engages and disengages with a mealtime schedule—life gets in the way! Shops regularly and has family meals a few times a week. Able to plan, shop, and cook meals.	Routine meals and snacks are established. The child knows what to expect. Parent is able to get back on track when obstacles (life!) occur.
Boundaries	Parent struggles with positive health behaviors; may have unaddressed past eating and body image concerns. The food environment is chaotic.	Parent sets limits but feels uncomfortable about saying "no." Child gets mixed messages about routines and boundaries.	Child understands the food routine, expectations, and limits. Feels secure in this environment.
Family Meals and Feeding Practices	Family gathers fewer than 3 times per week. Mealtime vibe includes pressure, criticism, or punishment. Incentives to eat, such as food rewards or catering, are used to get kids to eat. Food restriction may occur.	Mealtimes are happening with good weeks and not-so-good weeks. Some negative feeding practices exist, but parents are increasingly aware of the impact on the child and are experimenting with self-service meals.	Routine, pleasant family meals occur on a regular basis, at least 3–5 times per week. A variety of self-service and meal options are used. Parent promotes choice and autonomy at the table.

Lunchtime is over and your child pops into the kitchen an hour later and says, "I'm hungry! Can I have a snack?" Your response: "The kitchen is closed right now, sweetie. But we'll have a snack at three—let's get outside, it's such a nice day!" Here's why this works: You set a boundary, which reinforces the food routine you've built. You predict the future, or when your child will have a snack, building security and a sense of what to expect. Then, you divert their attention. Of course, the goal is a rhythmic routine, but there may be times when you have to go off schedule to meet your child's needs. That's okay.

Last, build your weekly schedule for family meals. How many family meals can you squeeze in? If dinner is a challenge, can you fit in a family breakfast or lunch during the week? Formalize your schedule and write it down. Next, determine what you will serve at the main meals. Sketch out what your meals could be. Pillar Six will provide more information on food balance and nutritious meals and snacks. Consider how you could serve them to optimize your child's autonomy. Family-style? Buffet? DIY? Build these into your weekly meal plan, as well. All you have to do is follow the plan.

Now, let's talk about the mealtime vibe. If you're a Learner, you might be feeling like you're doing mealtime all wrong. Talking too much about food or how well (or not) your child is eating. Reminder: stop talking about food, eating, health, nutrition, or anything that falls in line with these topics. Not only can this sour the family connection, but it can also be stigmatizing, especially if your child has a smaller or larger body. Nixing negative table talk will change the atmosphere almost instantly. What can you talk about instead? Your day, current events, future happenings, past occurrences, and family fun times.

Feeding practices, such as catering or incentivizing eating with dessert, pressure to eat, and food restriction, also need to go. Let me assure you, the only feeding "job" you have is to plan meals, make them, get them on the table, and keep the food atmosphere positive. That's it. (And that's plenty!) Remember, you don't have to get your child to eat. Eating is your child's "job." How freeing! If you tried my suggestions and still feel like you need more help in this area, a pediatric dietitian can be a great partner in helping you learn how to be more positive with feeding your child.

The Striver: Let's Level Up

Okay, you've got a routine down, are having family meals, and trying to avoid pressure, rewards, and catering. However, that old worry about your child's eating or their size comes back, and the negative feeding practices creep back in. Or unexpected changes happen, like a family illness, and they wipe out the schedule and routine you've established. Life happens. Remember: it's less about being rigid with schedules and routines and more about your flexibility and ability to bounce back and get back to the positive routines that are effective for your family. You're in this for the long game. Don't give up on family meals just because you had a bad week, went on vacation, or there was no schedule at all. Jump back in to the game as soon as possible.

If you're having three family meals each week, level up to four. Find another meal or snack during the week when your family can eat together. Get self-service meals on your weekly plan. Practice your boundaries. Say "not now" rather than "no"—you'll get more mileage and possibly less resistance. Remember, you're building security and supporting your child's appetite awareness. Your child will learn the routine.

The Thriver: Keep Up the Good Work

What can I say other than *Kudos!* Keep at it. As your child changes and grows, it's not uncommon to slip back to old, ineffective feeding tactics or loosen the structure or boundaries. It happens. Because you feed your child every day, *how* you do it will be an important cornerstone to their relationship with food. If things get hard, come back here to get on track.

Pull up a chair. Take a taste. Come join us.
Life is so endlessly delicious!

—RUTH REICHL

EATING

Tune In, Enjoy, and Avoid the "Blahs"

"The other day I lifted one of the couch cushions to find about fifteen empty bags of Pirate's Booty," shared Theresa, a mom from Connecticut. "Sadly, it wasn't even shocking to me. I'm worried for my daughter and don't know how to stop these habits before they become even harder to control." If you've ever wondered or worried about your child's eating—overindulging at a party, eating fast, being full after a few bites, or constantly talking about food—you're in the right place. Witnessing your child change their eating habits over the years, and not necessarily for the better, can make any parent get a little gray at the roots. But some of these eating changes are natural.

When I was a younger mother, I used to proudly state my goal as a parent was to raise children who could walk by a bowl of M&M'S or a plate of cookies, and take them or leave them. I believed that if my kids had a handle on their hunger and appetite, they would "eat for hunger." Boy, was I naive! Over the course of my career and motherhood, I've learned that children eat for a variety of reasons, some of which are not completely under their (or our) control. And some reasons have nothing to do with hunger.

Your child was born with the equipment and the mechanics to manage their eating. As a baby, they cried, fidgeted, fussed, and screamed to show they were hungry. They pulled away from the breast or bottle when they were full. They were masters of intuitive eating—eating from an awareness of their appetite and body sensations. As toddlers, they showed command of their appetite. They ate less (which you may have referred to as becoming "picky"), down-regulating in response to a slowing of their growth.

As kids grow, eating becomes complex. Your child no longer simply eats when they're hungry. They may eat when they're sad. When they're happy. When they're bored. When they want to. A combination of factors, including physiological and biological forces and emotional and psychological underpinnings, begins to influence their sense of appetite and their eating. It's idealistic to think kids will eat only when hungry, as it ignores the other influences at play, such as emotional regulation, executive functioning, feeding, distraction, and physical factors. There's a lot going on!

SCIENCE AND SOCIETY
Why Your Child Eats

A s a parent, much of what you do with food will end up influencing your child's food preferences and how they eat. If you serve lots of sweets and treats, for instance, your child may learn to prefer those foods. Likewise, if you serve and eat lots of fruits and vegetables and other nutritious foods, your child will grow to like those. You've learned that how you feed can change your child's eating, and not always for the better. Pressure to eat, restricting food access, or using food as a reward may heighten your child's sensitivity to food cues and lower their ability to interpret appetite signals.

Feeding kids is like a lesson in reverse psychology. Often, how you feed has the opposite effect on their eating. Attempts to control your child's food may cause more out-of-control eating. Pushing your child to eat results in more pushback from your child. Sweets become more charged and powerful when you use them as a reward or restrict them. And catering to your child's food requests keeps them wanting those same foods. And yet, within a family, each child and their eating habits are different. The good news is that children's eating habits *do* evolve over time, and you *do* have some influence. But you need to understand why your child eats first. Let's look at the four main reasons for eating: homeostasis, hedonism, executive functioning, and food approach.

Homeostasis: Eating to Achieve a State of Balance

Let me start by stating the obvious: we all need to eat to stay alive. Homeostasis, or the act of balancing the internal functions of the body's cells, organs, and tissues, relies on the energy that comes from food. When the body gets what it needs and everything is in balance, the body works well. Like a car, it hums along. Getting enough energy at the right time is primarily managed by your child's appetite, a complex system that includes hormones, the brain, the stomach and intestines, and a host of other players. Your child's appetite is what tells them when to eat, how much to eat, and when to stop eating.

The appetite control center is located in the brain. Hormones are sent as signals to trigger the sensation of hunger and fullness. As a result, when your child feels hungry, they feel a need to eat. When they feel full or satisfied, they slow eating and stop. Like a car that operates on gasoline, diesel, or electricity, the body uses food as its fuel. And like a gauge that tells you when your vehicle tank is full or empty, the brain, stomach, and certain hormones act together to tell the body when it needs more fuel or not. All of this is done to maintain homeostasis, or to keep the body balanced.

The hormones involved are called appetite hormones. There are many hormones that make up this complex appetite system, but for simplicity, I'll focus on two well-known appetite hormones: ghrelin and leptin. *Ghrelin* (pronounced "greh-luhn") is the hunger hormone. To remember this one easily, think, "Grrr, I'm hungry." Ghrelin is produced in the stomach and tells the brain it's time to eat. It's not only central to stimulating hunger, but it's also needed to release growth hormone. *Leptin* is the satiety, or fullness, hormone and is produced by fat cells. The more fat cells the body has, the more leptin is produced. Leptin helps your child stop eating when their body gets what it needs.

So what happens when your child's body is low on energy? The body releases ghrelin to trigger hunger and eating. Even in times of perceived starvation, like when a person diets or cuts calories to lose weight, the body will upregulate ghrelin to ensure the body gets enough energy. This process is biologically strong and nearly impossible to ignore. And it's often why those who lose weight may gain it back, and gain more. When your child eats enough food, leptin is triggered, cueing a sense of satisfaction or fullness. However, when a person has a lot of body fat, the brain may become *insensitive* to leptin, failing to perceive fullness completely, which can lead to overeating. Ideally, appetite hormones would govern our eating—we would eat when hungry and stop when full. But appetite isn't the only reason we eat.

WHY IS MY CHILD CONSTANTLY HUNGRY?

Some parents wonder why their child is always hungry, especially when they eat enough, are larger in size, or carry extra body fat. It has to do with *leptin resistance*. Abundant amounts of body fat lead the body to produce a lot of leptin. Instead of inducing fullness, though, too much leptin may cause leptin resistance. As a result, the feeling of fullness becomes muffled and dull. Stealthily, leptin also changes its behavior and *stimulates* appetite, rather than inducing fullness. This encourages more body fat and also lowers the number of calories being burned. Experts believe that a high amount of body fat, especially in the belly area, is a sign of leptin resistance. Can leptin resistance be reversed? The jury is still out on this. The catch-22 is that reducing body fat may trigger a starvation response that leads to more eating. This is why healthful lifestyle behaviors, including the Pillars of Wellness, are key to improving quality of life *and* physical health.

Hedonism: Wanting to Eat and the Pursuit of Pleasure

Have you ever eaten something simply because it looks too good to pass up? Or it brings back pleasant memories? Hedonic hunger describes the preoccupation with and desire to eat for the purpose of pleasure. It has nothing to do with hunger, homeostasis, or biological needs, and everything to do with reward. Eating is one of the most rewarding experiences of living, and it partly drives our motivation to eat. If we were controlled only by homeostatic eating, then eating would be like breathing or going to the bathroom—a necessary but unexciting part of our existence. In real life, everyone eats for need *and* for pleasure.

Unlike homeostatic eating, pleasure-based eating responds to *external* cues like the sight and smell of food. Looking forward to eating an ice-cream cone, remembering how good it tastes, and enjoying eating it, are hedonic messages that influence a desire to eat. When your child experiences pleasure while eating, it reinforces more eating. It's why they may overeat their favorite foods, palatable foods like cookies or chips, and foods they associate with positive memories or feelings.

What makes food and eating so enjoyable? The brain and its neurotransmitters. When food, especially flavors like sweet or salty, are consumed repeatedly, or there's a memory of a pleasurable experience, the release of dopamine and serotonin is triggered in the brain. Dopamine is a "feel-good" chemical, designed to keep us doing the things that ensure our survival, such as eating, drinking, and reproducing. When eating is pleasurable, the brain will anticipate and respond to food cues, increasing dopamine levels in the brain. In fact, the level of dopamine released is proportional to the amount of pleasure experienced. Sugary foods and those high in fat, for instance, have a powerful effect on the brain. They may blunt fullness cues, increase the length of a meal or snack, and stimulate the brain's reward system. This may lead to cravings and an increased desire to eat. However, over time, a phenomenon of "tolerance" unfolds, which is why eating an ice-cream cone every night after dinner becomes less rewarding.

Serotonin, the other neurotransmitter, is also a "feel-good" hormone and a mood stabilizer. About 10 percent of serotonin in the body is made in the brain—the rest is made in the intestines. Serotonin helps with digestion, increases the sense of fullness while eating, and may also suppress appetite in certain situations. Serotonin is made from the essential amino acid tryptophan, which we get from foods such as cheese, milk, and chicken. And, as described in Pillar Two, it's also the precursor to melatonin, which helps your child sleep. And yet there's another aspect behind why your child eats, and that's deciding to eat.

Executive Functioning: Deciding to Eat

Making a decision to eat or not rests on thinking and executive functioning skills. Executive functioning encompasses a range of skills, including decision-making, delayed gratification, inhibition, disinhibition, cognitive flexibility, and working memory. Executive functioning skills begin to develop in preschool and evolve throughout adolescence and beyond, helping your child make decisions about their behavior, including eating.

"I talk with my son before we head out to social events. I want him to be prepared for all the temptations there because he tends to lose control of his eating, especially when there's pizza," said Jillian, mom of a ten-year-old boy. "Sometimes this helps and other times he just can't stop." Making a decision in the moment is an example of an executive functioning skill. It involves taking in the information around you, remembering the plan or expectation, and deciding on an action. For children to be good at regulating their eating, they need to have executive functioning skills in the areas of inhibition, working memory, and cognitive flexibility.

Your child's behavior around food may be the best indicator of whether they'll eat a lot or not. For example, if you notice your child can't pass up sweets and treats or has a tendency to overeat in celebratory situations, it may be a sign that executive functioning skills are not fully developed. Children who are impulsive in other areas of their lives may have more difficulty controlling their behavior around tasty food and may benefit from having them less available. Preschoolers who can delay their gratification are better able to self-regulate eating and less likely to overeat than those who cannot. Last, children who are challenged in the area of cognitive flexibility or who demonstrate poor decision-making may gravitate toward higher-fat foods and sweets.

The Facets of Executive Function

Executive Skill	Explanation	Examples
Inhibition	The ability to show restraint when engaging with the world. Inhibition is considered a facet of temperament, like shyness around new people or unfamiliar places.	Child can decide to not eat cookies or chips. Child can take a reasonable amount of food rather than take most of what's offered, or choose when they'll eat dessert.
Disinhibition	A lack of restraint, or impulsivity.	May overeat when not hungry. May overeat in social situations where there is an abundance of food.
Working Memory	The small amount of information that can be held in the mind and used to perform tasks or make decisions.	Choosing to add a salad at lunch after learning about fruits and vegetables in class.
Delayed Gratification	The ability to put off an impulse or available reward in hopes of getting a more valuable reward in the future.	Child eats fruit at lunch, so they can have dessert at dinner. Child behaves at the doctor's office, so they can go to the toy store afterward.
Cognitive Flexibility	A child's ability to adjust behavior effectively and appropriately based on what's going on around them.	Able to roll with new, changed, or unplanned events, like not being able to get candy at the candy shop because it's closed for the day.

This is all to say that low executive functioning skills, especially impulsivity, poor inhibition, poor working memory, and cognitive inflexibility, may explain why some children eat too much. On the other hand, it's feasible that more body fat may cause physiological changes like increased inflammation and poor regulation of blood sugar and insulin, both of which may impair executive functioning. What does all this mean for your child? Poor or delayed executive functioning skills may influence your child's eating and be an area where more support is needed.

Approach to Food: Your Child's Natural Behavior

Aside from the biological reasons for eating, there are other reasons why children eat. Their eating style, for one. There are two main approaches to food: food avoidance and food responsiveness. *Food avoidance* is your child's sensitivity to being full after eating (also called satiety responsiveness). You can tell if your child is satiety responsive because they will slow their eating as they get full. *Food responsiveness*, on the other hand, is the enjoyment of food and a heightened sensitivity to food cues.

#TruthBomb: A food-responsive child may eat faster and consume more calories. A satiety-responsive child may consume fewer calories and eat slowly. These appetite traits are thought to be on a continuum, influencing each other.

Appetite traits are genetically inherited. In fact, food responsiveness is 59 percent heritable; food enjoyment is 53 percent heritable; satiety responsiveness is 72 percent heritable; and slowness in eating is 84 percent heritable. Interestingly, appetite traits have been measured in babies when the only food source they have is exclusively milk (breast milk or formula). Slowness in eating and enjoyment of food can be seen as early as *the first three months of life*, a sign that children are born with these traits.

Variations in appetite, according to studies in twins from birth on, suggest that food responsiveness at three months influences size at fifteen months, especially in situations where there are opportunities to eat. One study looked at the trajectory of growth based on food responsiveness or food avoidance behaviors and found that babies

The Spectrum of Appetite Traits in Children

Appetite Trait	What Is It?	Examples
Food Responsiveness	Desire for food after exposure to food cues, such as sight or smell; how aroused a child gets in response to food; how fast a child eats.	Child has a big appetite; asks for food often; would eat too much if allowed; can eat again after a meal or snack.
Enjoyment of Food	The reward of eating; the pleasure a child takes in eating.	Child loves food; interested in food; looks forward to mealtimes.
Satiety Responsiveness	A child's fullness threshold; a slowing of eating and a decrease in food intake after a meal or snack.	Child eats slowly, fills up quickly, leaves food on the plate after eating.
Slowness in Eating	The pace with which a child eats or finishes eating.	Child eats slowly; eats more and more slowly as the meal goes on; takes more than 30 minutes to eat a meal.
Fussiness	High selectivity over the range of foods that are acceptable to the child.	Child refuses new foods at first; dislikes a food without tasting it; is difficult to please with meals.
Emotional Overeating	Eats more food in response to negative emotional states, such as boredom or sadness.	Child eats more when worried, annoyed, anxious, or bored.
Emotional Undereating	Eats less food in response to negative emotions, such as stress or sadness.	Child eats less when upset, angry, or tired.
Desire to Drink	A constant urge to have a drink.	Child always has a drink with them, if allowed; always asking for a drink.

who were food responsive early in life grew more rapidly up to age fifteen months. Furthermore, other researchers have found connections between appetitive traits, especially a sensitivity to food cues and fullness, and body size.

"I've noticed lately that my daughter's appetite seems different than her siblings," said Hayley, mom to a five-year-old. "She gets emotional about food, feels hunger more intensely, and seems to think about it more." Differences in appetite traits and eating style may help explain why some kids are larger, and others smaller, even within the same family. There's a genetic heritability for body fat, but there are inherited appetite traits like food responsiveness, too, which may make some children more vulnerable to palatable and plentiful food, and prone to overeating. Just like children within a family may have different hair or eye color, or body size, kids can inherent different tendencies in their approach to food and eating.

Children who inherit an "avid appetite," who are "big eaters," or are more impulsive may be more tempted to eat when an abundance of tasty food is available. "Kids who are food responsive might have to activate their self-regulation, or executive functioning skills, to a greater degree to actually resist those tasty foods," says Dr. Alison Miller, a developmental psychologist at the University of Michigan School of Public Health and director of the Child Health and Development Lab. "As parents, it's important to keep in mind for some kids it might be harder to resist certain foods and take more work to do so." And remember the kids who fill up fast. They may eat slowly, become full earlier, and appear to be poor eaters. Although they may also be smaller in size, they may simply be more sensitive to fullness (satiety responsive). Overriding their appetite cues by urging them to eat more sets up a feeding dynamic that may be problematic down the road.

"My three-year-old daughter can eat as much for dinner as I do," said Deanna, a mom from Connecticut. "Honestly, I'm disturbed at how much she can eat. I worry she won't be able to stop . . . and what will that mean for her later as she grows up?" While your child's eating may be worrisome, I caution you: don't make appetite and eating a problem. These tendencies are built into your child, much like the tendency to be shy or outgoing. They're just one piece of the bigger, complex puzzle of eating. Making your child's eating a problem may make them ashamed, embarrassed, and prone to eating in secret and other unhelpful eating behaviors. Understanding the nuances around eating and the tendencies they embody will help you navigate what may be unsettling at times with sensitivity and understanding. Remember, children eat because their bodies need them to, they enjoy eating, they decide to eat, and they have inherent traits and eating styles that encourage their behaviors.

Takeaways:

- The reasons for eating are complex and include biological, psychological, emotional, and genetic foundations.

- To regulate eating well, children need appetite awareness and good executive functioning skills in the areas of inhibition, working memory, and cognitive flexibility.

- A child's behavior around food may be an indicator of whether they will eat enough, too much, or not enough.

OBJECTIONS AND OBSTACLES:
Too Much Eating (Or Not Enough)

The answer to "Why does my child eat like this?" isn't straightforward, as you can see. Your child is governed by appetite cues, pleasure, the ability to manage food in a variety of contexts, their genetic makeup, eating style, and other factors. Plus, there are obstacles inherent in the world in which they live. It's a lot to navigate! In this section we'll explore the emotional and external factors that influence eating, including stress, emotions, and eating when not hungry. These may lead to unhelpful eating patterns and impact both physical health and emotional well-being.

Stress and Eating

Stress is a powerful influence on eating. When stressed or threatened, your child's brain activates the release of cortisol (the primary stress hormone) and adrenaline. Cortisol increases blood sugar and activates its use in the brain, while down-regulating nonessential activities in the body. Adrenaline raises heart rate and blood pressure. The uptick in these hormones spurs the "fight, flight, or freeze" reaction. If your child is regularly stressed or threatened, the stress response is constantly engaged. Long-term activation of cortisol can mess up almost every biological process in the body, including increasing the risk of anxiety, depression, digestive problems, sleep problems, poor appetite regulation, and more. Stress alone may trigger eating behaviors. Chronic stress may stimulate the hunger hormone and dull the sense of fullness, both of which lower motivation, cause moodiness, and encourage eating to take the edge off of stress. "Foods that are high in sugar, fat, and salt are biologically soothing to us," says Miller.

> **#TruthBomb:**
> Children who wake up with high cortisol levels or who experience acute stress secrete more salivary cortisol, which is associated with eating more sweet and fatty foods.

Emotional Eating

When your child feels discomfort, stress, or negative emotions, they may look for relief, and that can be through eating. Because food itself and eating are pleasurable and comforting experiences, both can create a sense of calm and good feeling. Some children turn to food when they experience any kind of stress, such as the pressure of taking exams or difficult peer relationships. Other kids may turn away from food when stress is present. Just like the adult who cannot eat when anxious about work, or who overeats when relationships are on the rocks, children, too, may respond to stress and emotions by eating, or not, to help them cope. Children who turn to food when they experience feelings of rejection, anxiety, loneliness, boredom, or negative emotions may be emotionally eating. When food provides comfort, however, it may help your child get through a challenging time, and that can be productive. But if your child relies on eating as a consistent way to deal with their emotions, it can turn into an unhelpful coping mechanism.

Of course, both *why* kids eat and *what* kids eat influence their later health outcomes. Eating to soothe emotions may center on sweet and savory foods, and the possibility for overeating is high. Studies suggest that children between the ages of six and fourteen years lose control of their eating about 2–10 percent of the time, globally, and children with larger bodies, 15–37 percent of the time. Kids who are smaller may experience heightened satiety responsiveness as a result of negative emotions, leading to less eating. Especially in children who are selective eaters, early satiety contributes to poor or inadequate eating, nutritional deficiencies, and slowed growth.

THE GROWING PREVALENCE OF DISORDERED EATING

The pressures to fit in—be slim, fit, and attractive—lead some children down the path of disordered eating. In children, this can show up initially as an effort to eat healthier, such as nixing carbs, sweets, or eating only "whole" foods. But this can turn into more rigid and restrained ways of eating, or a loss of control with eating, like yo-yoing between eating "healthy" during the daytime and binging at night. A recent global meta-analysis reported 20 percent of six- to eighteen-year-olds show signs of dysfunctional eating behaviors. Girls had a higher prevalence (30 percent) than boys (17 percent), and children with larger bodies demonstrated more disordered eating as they got older if their bodies grew in size.

The BLAHS and Eating When Not Hungry

Have you ever noticed that your child eats when bored? Or says they're hungry right after having a meal? Or maybe you've noticed secret eating. They may have the BLAHS, an acronym that stands for *Boredom, Loneliness, Avoidance, Habit, and Situation*, which makes up some of the common reasons for eating when not hungry. *Boredom* is a state of

EATING IN THE ABSENCE OF HUNGER (EAH)

Eating in the absence of hunger (EAH) describes continued eating despite fullness, or for reasons other than hunger. Children who eat without hunger are less able to self-regulate their energy intake and are more vulnerable to eating sweets and treats despite feeling satisfied after eating. EAH was reported in girls between the ages of five and seven years in 1999. Today, and for a variety of reasons, children *as young as eighteen months* are susceptible to EAH, especially in contexts where there is an opportunity to eat.

having nothing to do, feeling disinterested, or feeling that life is dull. *Loneliness* is a state of, or feeling of, isolation. *Avoidance* means turning away or detaching from emotions. The emotions are there, but the child may internalize and avoid feelings such as anger, disappointment, or sadness, for instance. *Habit* is a regular practice, which can be helpful or not, such as eating at the table (a good habit) or sneaking into the pantry when parents aren't around (an unhelpful habit). Habits are ingrained behaviors that occur without thought. *Situation* is the environmental context that supports eating when not hungry. For example, an abundance of minimally nutritious snacks in the home or at a party may place some kids in a tempting environment that's too hard to pass up. When children have the BLAHS they may turn to food, eating to pass the time, to chase away uncomfortable feelings, or as an automatic response. Boredom, particularly, is a predictor of emotional eating. The problem with the BLAHS is that your child may disregard their appetite cues and eat beyond fullness.

The Mouthwatering Food Environment

What's in the kitchen, and how easy it is to grab and eat, affects what your child actually ends up eating. Simply said, some kids will pass up the bowl of M&M'S because they're not hungry, and others won't be able to. They'll dive in for reasons beyond hunger. The presence of cookies, chips, and candy may be too much for kids who are food responsive. Access to sweets or savory foods may challenge executive functioning skills, drive the reward pathway, and be the go-to when kids have the BLAHS. While food restriction may cause a scenario of scarcity, triggering a desire to seek and eat food, the opposite is true as well. Abundant, easy-to-access tasty foods may be too inviting for some kids to stay away from. No doubt, this is complicated!

#WiseAdvice:
Precision food parenting—a diplomatic style, responsiveness, and an eye on the innate tendencies of your child—will be key to supporting them as you cultivate good eating habits.

"My son is driven to eat," relayed Jasmine. "He's triggered by food, has ADHD and is impulsive, and talks about food all the time." During the pandemic, Jasmine's twelve-year-old son gained thirty pounds. She consulted a dietitian who encouraged Jasmine to make sweets and treats more available as a way to remove their power and draw. "I really wanted this to work for my son, but unfortunately, it was too unstructured," she reported. "He put on more weight, and I feel like we have more struggles with food." There's no pat solution or one-size-fits-all advice for children and their eating. One child may need more structure and less temptation, while another may need more flexibility and food availability. There's nuance. The real answer is to be curious about your child's eating, appreciate the underlying influences, and attempt to set them up for success knowing that you may have to make some adjustments if things aren't working.

Understanding your child's eating tendencies and reasons for eating is key to helping them become good eaters. While the structure, boundaries, and routines you learned about in the last Pillar help a lot, it's also true that each child will be different. If you're dealing with multiple children in the family who have different eating styles, or who have challenges with executive functioning or impulsivity, helping them without food restriction or too much temptation is the key. "Just like you would keep an extra eye on your impulsive child who might run out into the road, you may need to monitor the food environment and tailor it to your child's appetitive traits," says Dr. Miller. Thankfully, there are strategies you can try to help everyone in the family be better regulated with eating. That's where we'll go next.

Takeaways:

- Stress may encourage eating, dull the sense of fullness, or turn off eating.

- Emotional eating and eating due to the BLAHS may be tools for coping with negative emotions and boredom. Done too much, they can be barriers to good eating habits.

- Food environments where palatable foods are plentiful may be harder for kids who are inherently more responsive to them.

HOW TO STRIVE AND THRIVE
Self-Regulation Is the Goal

"My child has always been in a larger body, is active most days, and eats more than I do," wrote Lindsey, mom to a seven-year-old girl. "Sometimes it just seems like she sees food, or thinks about it, and wants to eat. Are children really able to know their hunger and fullness cues?" Given inborn appetite traits, the food environment, food restriction, food permissiveness, and balancing all foods in a nutritious diet, it can be easy to forget that eating should be a nurturing, joyful experience. Let me reassure you: your child has what it takes to tune in to their bodily sensations and self-regulate their eating. And they have the right to enjoy food. Awareness and enjoyment are allies in establishing good eating habits. But if your child faces specific challenges with eating, you'll want to support them in the best way possible (and avoid the feeding mistakes that can complicate the matter). Even if your child is a good eater, the following advice will mitigate stress by keeping them tuned into their appetite and body sensations, and keep them focused on eating for need and pleasure.

I'll discuss mindfulness and mindful eating, and offer you language and conversation starters to help your child identify how they feel when eating, when hungry, and when they have the BLAHS. We'll also explore what to do about food triggers and temptations in the eating environment. The goal here is to encourage your child to be more aware of their appetite, create a food environment that supports them, and emphasize food enjoyment.

Paying Attention When Eating

Mindful eating, or tuning into the process of and sensations felt during eating, helps children pay attention to their appetite. It may involve pausing between bites, chewing food thoroughly, or noticing the characteristics of food, like appearance, texture, or odor. When TV, phones, or games join your child at the table, it's harder for them to pay

A MINDFUL EATING EXPERIMENT

Here's a way to introduce the concept of mindful eating and engage your child in identifying their sensations around food and eating, versus simply ingesting food in a mindless, hurried fashion. Take a Hershey's Kiss or a piece of candy like Skittles. Have your child eat the candy the way they normally do. They can take a pause and drink some water. Then, give them another piece of the same candy and take them through the following series of steps, allowing time between each step:

1. **Hold the candy.** Notice how it feels in your fingers or palm.

2. **See it.** Let your eyes notice all the details. What do you see?

3. **Touch it.** Explore the texture. What does it feel like?

4. **Smell it.** Notice the fragrance. What is happening in your tummy?

5. **Place it on the tongue.** Don't chew it! Let it melt there. Notice what this feels like.

6. **Taste it.** What is the flavor? Is it changing as it melts?

7. **Swallow it.** How do you know it's time to swallow?

8. **Follow it.** How does it feel when the candy moves down your throat and into your body?

attention to eating and the sensations that occur within their bodies. Distractions dilute the ability to be mindful.

Mindful eating may improve appetite regulation, lower stress, counteract unhelpful eating patterns, and help your child develop a greater appreciation of food. If too much enjoyment of food drums up visions of overeating, rest assured. It turns out that when kids enjoy what they eat, they're more likely to feel satisfied and more likely to make food choices that benefit their health.

Mindfulness Helps Stress and Emotions, Too

Mindfulness, in general, is a way to moderate stress. It's especially helpful in protecting your child from mental health conditions like anxiety and depression. So how do you practice mindfulness? For young children, doing arts and crafts, drawing or coloring, and working on puzzles in a quiet environment can calm the nervous system. Using breath and breathing, such as belly breathing or rainbow breathing (see box below), to calm down and be more mindful can reduce stress levels. Movement, being outside in nature, journaling, yoga, and meditation are effective, too.

BREATHING TO CALM DOWN

Breathing helps calm the nervous system and increases mindfulness. Here are a couple of techniques:

Belly Breathing: Have your child lie down on their back and place a stuffed animal on their belly. Tell them to breathe in and move the animal up, hold for three or four seconds; breathe out and bring the animal back down while counting to three or four. This technique teaches your child to take deep breaths using their belly.

Rainbow Breathing: Your child stands with their arms at the sides of their body. Instruct them to inhale and raise their arms overhead like a rainbow, then exhale and lower them. Encourage your child to go slowly.

Kids have all kinds of emotions, but they don't necessarily understand them. Our society encourages us to "grin and bear" difficulties, but this is a disservice to kids and may disconnect them from their feelings. Instead, help your child identify them. Give them the words to describe how they're feeling, such as sad, lonely, disappointed, frustrated, angry, lost, content, or happy. Let them claim those feelings without shame.

Pretend play can be a way to help children sort out their feelings. When your younger child is feeding their baby doll, you can say, "Dolly needs to eat. What should we do?" Or when you play chef in the kitchen, "Chef is having a dinner party. What should we make?" As the play begins, listen for opportunities to talk about how the baby feels (hungry, full, cranky) or how the chef is managing the pressures of cooking for a crowd (stressed out, distracted, excited).

Emotion coaching, or the practice of helping your child be in touch with their emotions and cope with them, is something you can do every day and is helpful for negative emotions like anger, sadness, or fear. If you get hung up on what to say about eating behaviors, I encourage you to remain calm and treat them like you would any other behavior that warrants calm parenting. Avoid problematizing eating. Rather, view your child's eating on a spectrum where eating behaviors and their variations are normal and not necessarily leading to poor health or habits. Here are some suggested responses to help you coach your child:

- When your child asks for food and you say no, say, *"I know you want [xyz food] right now, but that's not what we're having today. We can have that on [upcoming day of the week]."*

- When they throw a tantrum because you're not serving their favorite foods, say, *"I can see you're upset. That's okay. You have big feelings, but it's not okay to [scream, hit me, or other negative action]. Let's cuddle on the couch with a book."*

- When your child is angry because you say no to sweets and treats, say, *"It's okay to be mad/disappointed about [not having cookies for snack time today]. Tomorrow's another day, and we can have some then."*

- When you catch your child sneaking, hiding, or engaging in another food-related misbehavior, say, *"Let's pause, collect ourselves, talk about this, and make a plan together."*

WHAT IS INTUITIVE EATING?

Intuitive eating, an approach to eating developed by dietitians Evelyn Tribole and Elyse Resch, integrates appetite awareness, instinct, emotions, and thinking, and promotes trusting the body in deciding what and how much to eat. Practicing intuitive eating attempts to regain the innate awareness of what the body needs and counteract the damage of diet culture. Adults who guide their eating using intuitive eating principles have the following commonalities: They don't overthink food or dieting, nor do they ignore their hunger cues. They don't categorize foods as "good" or "bad," but rather select foods for enjoyment and optimal body function. They respect their hunger and fullness cues, eating when hungry and stopping when full or satisfied. They are more likely to have positive body image, self-esteem, and well-being, and less likely to binge eat or lose control of eating. They don't restrict, diet, or follow food rules like "no carbs." They're also less likely to be emotional eaters, eat in response to external triggers, or have an unhealthy focus on their size or shape. Children are naturally intuitive at birth, but many factors can change this as they grow, leaving them more sensitive to external cues for eating. If you're curious to learn more about intuitive eating, check out my resources in the Appendix.

- When your child is eating due to the BLAHS, or using food to calm themselves, say, *"I see you're upset. I believe you, and I'm here to support you. What's going on?"*

Talking About Appetite, Eating, and Food

Young children are pretty good at appetite awareness, but studies show that as they grow up, they become less attuned to what their bodies tell them about eating. That's because external factors begin to override internal sensations. You can help your child be in touch with their physical and emotional needs around eating through everyday conversation. In the most basic sense, you'll want to start talking about appetite cues very early on. Toddlers know when their bellies are hungry and when they're full. You can use terms like "hungry belly" and "happy belly." Keep it simple. You can ask them things like *What's your tummy telling you? Is your tummy happy? Does your belly need more?* Remember, toddlers and preschoolers have developing cognitive skills. They need simplification. When the belly is growling, feels empty, and hasn't had food for a while, help them associate this with hunger. Responding appropriately to this cue also reinforces your child's ability to recognize it. When your child seems satisfied, is slowing down, is distracted, or refuses more food, these are signs of fullness. Your child has a "happy belly." Again, ending a meal when your child shows fullness helps them stay aware of this signal. It's natural to focus on hunger more than satisfaction or fullness—as parents, we feel uncomfortable when our kids have real (or perceived) hunger—but it's important to focus on *both* appetite cues. From my observation, kids are less sensitive to feeling full than they are to sensing hunger, so help them recognize this distinction.

When your child is older, you can have deeper conversations. You can ask *How does your body tell you it's hungry? What does it feel like? What does it feel like when your tummy is getting full?* Talking about these sensations will bring your child greater awareness of what's going on inside. You can also talk about food and the environmental cues that prompt a desire to eat or stop eating: *What do you love about that food? How does your body feel when you see all that food at the party? What is it about [xyz] food that turns you off?*

Also consider your child's state. Are they emotional, excited, or bored? A child's state may inform their eating behavior. Observe with curiosity and without judgment. *I notice when you're stressed about homework, you [eating behavior]. What's happening in your body then?* Or *You seem bored. What are you feeling?*

Last, acknowledge that your child may not get enough exposure to certain foods, like sweets, which may spur unhelpful eating behaviors. And let's not forget, your child may have wonderful memories of food, or sheer enjoyment of certain foods, flavors, and eating. If your child loves food and enjoys eating, celebrate! It's a good thing to desire and enjoy the very thing that sustains life. The goal here is to help your child understand their

#WiseAdvice: Give your child permission to eat, because anything less may feed them shame and trigger dysfunctional eating behaviors.

WHAT IS UNCONDITIONAL PERMISSION TO EAT?

U nconditional permission to eat means you give your child the green light to eat and enjoy all foods while removing the moral judgment about them. This encourages a relaxed relationship and combats guilt and shame when eating indulgent foods, or eating too much or too little food. Unconditional permission to eat does not replace your feeding strategy, structure, or routines, but it does nix moral and virtuosic values about eating a certain way.

body's needs, wants, and desires, and navigate them in ways that support and sustain both physical health and emotional well-being.

Other Ways to Interpret Appetite Sensations

Older children, due to their developmental stage, may be better able to interpret their hunger and fullness when they see a scale of appetite sensations. An appetite scale is like a pain scale that gauges the spectrum of pain from one to ten. Keep this simple. On the scale ranging from hunger to fullness, a "one" is painfully hungry/starving; a "five" is ambivalent (neither hungry nor full); and a "ten" is uncomfortable, bursting full.

Another way to help your child understand their eating is to run through the BLAHS Test, which may support their appetite awareness

THE BLAHS TEST

Are you bored? Let's find something to do.

Are you lonely? Let's connect.

Are you having feelings or emotions about something? Let's talk.

Is this a habit? Let's reprogram.

Is this situation triggering you? Let's relocate or reframe.

and self-regulation. You can do a quick BLAHS check-in with a series of questions that address the most common reasons kids eat when they're not hungry. The spirit of this exercise is to be light, positive, curious, and nonstigmatizing.

These exercises are designed to help you open up the conversation about eating and help your child recognize eating patterns for themself. If any of these tools don't feel right, then move on.

Triggers, Temptations, and Training for Better Regulation

As you've learned, some kids will naturally be more aroused by food or impulsive around it. If you know your child has these built-in tendencies, there are several ways you can help. One way is through *self-regulation training.* For example, if your child is a fast eater, you can help by teaching them to slow down using a technique called Take 5. Have your child put the fork or utensil down after taking a bite of food. Ask them to close their eyes, breathe, and count to five on one hand for each breath. This slowing-down technique is also useful for the child who has difficulty recognizing when they're full. Just putting the fork down or taking a sip of water between bites can slow down a fast eater and allow the child who's unsure about their fullness to sense it.

For children who are more aroused by food cues, another strategy is to limit the availability of sweets and treats. I caution you here, though. Restricting food can blur the situation, as some kids will be more drawn to foods that are controlled. I encourage you to carefully watch your child's response if you limit palatable foods. Some kids will turn into food seekers, perhaps raiding the pantry, sneaking food, or hiding it. However, if your child is naturally food-responsive, having more structure in the kitchen, like scheduling predictable access to tempting foods, may help curtail food responses.

Last, be respectful of the child who demonstrates early satiety or who is sensitive to fullness. While they may eat better with more frequent offerings of food, you still want to keep them engaged with their appetite cues and tuned into their bodies, rather than push them to have a bigger appetite.

THE WHOLE-CHILD CHECKUP
Eating

N   ow that you're more informed about your child's eating, let's check in and explore how you can grow. First, let's identify whether you're a Learner, Striver, or Thriver.

The Learner: Where Do I Begin?

If you identify as a Learner, getting a better understanding of your child's eating style is the first step. Do they have a good sense of hunger, or are they relying on external cues to eat? Are they impulsive around food? Do they eat (or not) based on feelings or negative emotions? Are they triggered by sweets and treats (remember, if these have been scarce or controlled, temptation for them may be higher), or sensitive to fullness? It's helpful to understand their appetitive traits. To build more awareness, have conversations about eating by using some of the questions outlined earlier. Keep it age-appropriate. Sharing your own experiences and sensations of food, appetite, and eating may help you open up the conversation with your child.

Experiment with mindful eating. Do the exercise outlined earlier on page 132, changing it up with different foods and timing. Make it fun and see where it takes you. If you notice you've got a fast eater, try the Take 5 exercise described on the previous page. The goal is to work on mindful eating practices in your home on a regular basis.

Assess your food environment. In an interview on my podcast with Dr. Lori Fishman, a child psychologist from Boston, she points out, "If you know your child really struggles with sweets, you don't have to bake cookies and leave them out on the counter, and then get mad at them for taking them." Instead, set up a food environment that supports your child and doesn't feed into any struggle they may have with eating. If you know chips will disappear, then you don't need to buy them often. And, if you do have them around, don't attach conditions to eating them, like eating vegetables or a certain amount of food. Work them into your food plan (more on that in the next Pillar). Set your child up for success by making positive modifications in your environment that will assist your child. A pediatric dietitian can hold your hand through this process!

Eating: Learner, Striver, or Thriver

	Learner	Striver	Thriver
Mindfulness and Mindful Eating	Emotions run high around food; child seems "obsessed" with food, compulsive with eating; eats fast, overeats, or eats when bored. Parent may also be overly responsive to food cues or may use food to soothe. Distractions are present at mealtime.	Aware of eating tendencies in child and self. Beginning to help child work through these with emotion coaching, mindful eating, and mindfulness techniques. Fewer distractions present while eating.	Encourages mindfulness and mindful eating practices. No distractions during meals or snacks. Child is sensitive to appetite cues, eats when hungry, stops when full. Enjoys food and eating.
Building Appetite Awareness Through Communication	Little conversation about appetite and eating. Parents are unsure how to respond when child is undereating, overeating, or demonstrating other troubling eating behaviors. Talking about food and eating feels uncomfortable.	Learning about and beginning to talk about appetite cues and feelings; coaching child through various emotions, triggers, and temptations around food. Parent may be sorting through their own experiences with food and eating.	Family has open, nonjudgmental dialogue about appetite, food, and eating; child has unconditional permission to eat. Child talks about hunger, fullness, emotions, and feelings. Child is learning to self-regulate eating in a variety of environments.
Food Temptations and Triggers	Presence of palatable foods creates food struggles between child and parent. Parent unaware of child's innate tendencies toward food, and views them as intentional behaviors.	Aware of child tendencies with eating, parent creates a supportive food environment. Occasionally uses counterproductive feeding, especially when tempting foods are around.	Food environment is flexible but not overly tempting. Parent keenly aware of child's eating style and aims to create food enjoyment alongside an environment that doesn't cause unnecessary struggle.

The Striver: Let's Level Up

Maybe you've experimented with mindful eating or already understand appetite cues, mindfulness, positive communication about eating, and the food environment that supports your child's eating style and tendencies. That's awesome! Take this opportunity to reevaluate what's going well, where you might be getting stuck, and where you can press forward.

Do you need to hone your emotion-coaching skills to better navigate conversations around food? Are you facing struggles yourself with eating? Are hard-to-resist foods accumulating in the kitchen, making it harder for your child? Take inventory and make a plan to move forward. No blame. No shame. Just harness that willingness to improve and shape your child's eating habits with understanding and sensitivity.

Practice mindful eating. If distractions like phones or TV during mealtimes are creeping in, reset the balance. Look for neutral, nonstigmatizing, teachable moments about appetite, eating, and food triggers. The goal is to help your child get to know themself better, be appetite- and emotion-articulate, build eating habits that nourish and nurture them, and emphasize the joy of eating.

The Thriver: Keep Up the Good Work

Congrats! Having good eating habits means understanding one's appetite, responding appropriately, avoiding food as a routine coping mechanism for emotions or the BLAHS, and being more mindful when eating. The hard thing will be facing the forces that will inevitably challenge your child's eating behaviors as they grow up, like more independence in the teen years. But, hey, you can navigate this!

One cannot think well, love well,
sleep well, if one has not dined well.

—VIRGINIA WOOLF

FOOD

Fluency and a
Flexible Balance

"My five-year-old says she is always hungry," said Renee. "She would snack all day if she could." As in Renee's case, frustrations with children may center on food. When it comes to a child's health, parents have a lot of questions, especially about food. After all, you engage with it all day and appreciate the connection between food and health. When *any* child is making less-than-nutritious food choices, watching them do so can be troubling. But at the same time, you want your child to enjoy food and the treats and eating experiences that go with childhood.

I believe our society places too much emphasis on food, giving it more power than it deserves. You've heard "food is medicine," but is it? Sure, a nutritious diet offers a variety of nutrients that are important for your child's growth and development and contributes to their longevity and health. No argument here. But when we attach moral virtue to food, it puts food in a boxing match, where one food is either *healthy* or *toxic, good* or *bad, natural* or *processed junk*, and there's only one winner. "Food is medicine" implies if you feed your child "healthy food" they will be healthy. But this may suggest that food can cure chronic diseases, or that if your child has developed an illness you've caused it. A continuum lies between "healthy" and "unhealthy," and that's where many families like yours and mine live, trying to create meals that are pleasing while promoting health and enjoyment. Oftentimes, the glorification of food ignores an important reality—that cost, flavor, availability, effort, and enjoyment matter quite a bit in our food decisions.

Food is both nourishment and nurturance for all children. All children need to eat an adequately nutritious diet in an environment that is nurturing. Food is key to every child's quality of life and enjoyment. The good news is there's no right or wrong diet. You can be *really* flexible about food. You don't have to be strict about an uber-healthy diet and avoid every treat, indulgence, or packaged food. There is a way to balance food so your child gets the nourishment they need, enjoys eating, and grows up healthy. And I believe it has to do with making food less complicated.

> **#TruthBomb:** The idea that children who are larger or smaller need different foods is archaic and a form of sizeism.

The goal of this Pillar is to teach you how to be food fluent and flexible so you can capitalize on nutrition, satisfaction, and enjoyment, without being overly concerned or frustrated. You'll learn how to plan meals and snacks so they're balanced, nutritious, and satisfying, and avoid the pitfalls of minimally nutritious foods and food shaming. Let's get started!

SCIENCE AND SOCIETY
Become Food Fluent

Children have more exposure to food than ever before, and this undoubtedly makes it harder for parents to strike a food balance that feels right, especially for their health. "My daughter, who is nine, is a picky eater," wrote Joy. "I always offer something 'safe' at every meal, but the food I prepare (whole foods cooking) is rejected constantly; I worry about her nutrition so much." When you have a child who won't eat or who prefers sweets and treats above all else, providing a nutritious diet can become hard and complicated. Let's reverse that and start with the basics: what food does for your child, and how to keep it satisfying and uncomplicated.

Food, Simplified

Food is complicated—more than it needs to be. From "healthy" to "processed," and everything in between (and there's a lot!), we've developed ideologies about food that make it trickier to feed kids, or at least feel good about it. In my thirty-plus-year career, I'd say a "healthy" diet is harder to define, influenced by underlying social biases, economic structures, and the nuances around what "healthy" means for every individual. In other words, what is "healthy" for me may not be "healthy" for you, and vice versa. I'm going to try to simplify things. Of course, some foods are more nutritious than others, but there's a role for *all* foods and your child can learn about them. Ideally, without prejudice, bias, or shame.

The calories, macronutrients (proteins, fats, and carbohydrates), and micronutrients (vitamins and minerals) from food are the fuel that helps your child's body grow and develop and keeps their "engine" running. A nutrient-rich diet is a goal for *every* person as it supports and promotes health and prevents disease. It includes a balance of fruits, vegetables, whole grains, lean sources of protein, dairy foods, and fats, also known as the food groups, and lower amounts of saturated fat, salt, and added sugar.

But kids don't need a perfect diet to grow well. Adequate nutrition is the goal. You can get this from a blend of different foods, including highly nutritious foods and minimally nutritious foods, and everything in between. Certainly, missing out on critical nutrients or getting too much of others can compromise health, growth, and body functioning. But treating food like a test you have to ace to be a successful parent, or minimizing food to a plate of nutrients, negates the joy of eating (and feeding), and perpetuates a food hierarchy that may lead to guilt and a weird relationship with food.

The nutrients in food are the key to unlocking its increasing complexity. Food can be *highly nutritious, decently nutritious,* or *minimally nutritious* based on the types and amounts of nutrients it contains. (I've written ad nauseam about food groups and eating plans in my other books, so for this Pillar, I'm simplifying things even more.) *Highly nutritious foods* are packed with nutrients your child needs every day. Conventionally, we think of these as categories of food, also known as the food groups (protein, dairy, fruits, vegetables, grains, and fats and oils). These are emphasized by the Dietary Guidelines for Americans (DGA) as the foundation of your child's eating pattern. *Decently nutritious foods* also have a lot of nutrients but contain other elements, like more fat and sugar. Sugary cereal, sweetened yogurt, and chicken nuggets come to mind. They contribute important nutrients but may be more appealing to your child due to their sweetness or savory flavor. *Minimally nutritious foods* offer few nutrients and are mostly sugar, fat, and salt. These tasty foods, such as cookies, chips, candy, french fries, and sugary drinks, have a high appeal and offer enjoyment to children.

In all, kids eat a range of foods. Sometimes they like foods that aren't always regarded as good for them, and dislike those that are, which can be frustrating. Diet culture would have you believe that only highly nutritious foods are worthy, but in truth, all types of foods can fit in and contribute to a balanced diet, whether they add a good source of nutrients or increase the pleasure of eating. One day of eating doesn't make or break the health of your child. It's the overall balance that will. The goal isn't to have a highly nutritious diet *all* the time, but

HOW HEALTHFULLY ARE KIDS EATING?

A snapshot of kids' eating patterns, measured by the Healthy Eating Index (HEI), a scoring metric that evaluates overall diet quality compared to the goals outlined by the 2020 DGA, reveals that toddlers aged two to four have a poor diet quality, demonstrated by an HEI score of 61 (0–100 range, with 100 being a diet of excellent quality). From here, the HEI score gets *worse* as children age, with kids aged five to eight having a score of 55 and kids aged nine to thirteen scoring a 52. What contributes to these low scores? A lack of highly and decently nutritious foods, and too many minimally nutritious foods.

to combine all types of foods so that your child gets *adequate* nutrition and is able to enjoy the foods they eat. If going for a highly nutritious diet makes you restrict, control, or freak out about minimally nutritious foods, or even packaged, decently nutritious foods, then I urge you to keep reading. You will learn about balancing all foods, being flexible, and becoming food fluent.

Highly Nutritious Foods

Have you ever listened to a choir or an a capella group? They're made up of a mix of different voices—tenor, baritone, bass, contralto, soprano. Together, they make a beautiful sound.

Similarly, the food groups can be combined to make a nutritious meal or snack. Each food group comprises foods with a concentrated source of similar nutrients. For example, foods rich in calcium are lumped together in the dairy group and iron-rich foods are mostly found in the protein group. Food groups may include food sourced from the land (fresh vegetables, whole grains, fresh fruit, meats, and other protein foods, for instance), or from a box, can, or bag (pasta, bread, tuna, beans, cereal). Just because it's in a package doesn't mean it's not nutritious.

EXAMPLES OF FOODS IN THE FOOD GROUPS

Protein Group: Meats, eggs, seafood, nuts and nut butter, legumes and peas, soy foods

Grain Group: Bread, crackers, cereal, pasta, rice, grits, and tortillas

Dairy Group: Milk, yogurt, cheese, and calcium-fortified soymilk

Fruit Group: Apples, frozen berries, canned peaches, raisins, and 100 percent orange juice

Vegetable Group: Tomatoes, carrots, spinach, lettuce, potatoes, corn, beans, cauliflower

Fats and Oils Group: Butter, olive oil, nuts, avocado, olives

Food groups provide a framework for planning, creating, and providing a balance of highly nutritious foods in your child's diet. Whether you're serving eggs and toast for dinner or chicken and rice, you're serving foods from the protein and grain groups, netting similar nutrients even though the actual foods are different. Now that's flexibility! In other words, combining different foods from the groups increases the overall nutrients and nutrition your child gets. You can find more in-depth information about the food groups at MyPlate, the nutrition guide published by the USDA's Center for Nutrition Policy and Promotion.

Decently Nutritious Foods

Decently nutritious foods may have added sugar, salt, or fat, but they still contribute a good source of nutrients. Think about cereal, granola bars, sweetened yogurt, canned soups, or boxed macaroni and cheese. Yes, there's the presence of added sugar, salt, or fat, but there are also meaningful amounts of nutrients that are good for your child. This can feel like no-man's-land and a slippery slope, especially if you've been sensitized to the mainstream messaging pitting foods against each other. Remember, nearly everything we eat must be processed, so it's ready for safe consumption. Even milk, yogurt, meats, pasta, canned fruit, and frozen vegetables all get some level of processing so they can be packaged, shelved, transported safely, and made ready for consumption. With decently nutritious foods, the key is in the balance of nutrient content. Diet culture and wellness gurus may make you feel guilty about offering them (and minimally nutritious foods), but the reality is decently nutritious foods may increase the nutrient content of the diet, and they are affordable, accessible, and taste good—common reasons why parents purchase them and their children eat them.

Minimally Nutritious Foods

Minimally nutritious foods are items like snack foods and desserts. They supply few key nutrients but offer higher amounts of fat, salt, and sugar. Desserts such as cookies, cakes, cupcakes, brownies, and candy; sugary drinks; and fried foods like french fries or chips are examples. Of course, minimally nutritious foods are quite tasty. There's room for them in your child's diet, and they can provide a source of enjoyment.

Nutrients Are the Key

Overall, your child needs a variety of nutrients each day to support their growth and development. Many nutrients are found together in foods, such as calcium and vitamin D in dairy foods or protein, iron, and zinc in protein foods like meat and beans. This is good news! Focusing on highly nutritious and decently nutritious foods (aka the food groups) will help your child get the nutrients they need. The table on page 150 highlights some of the key nutrients and what they do for your child.

How do you know if a food is highly, decently, or minimally nutritious? And how do you translate this to everyday eating? By looking at food through what I call a "nutrient lens." A nutrient lens allows you to determine whether a food will contribute nutritionally to your child's diet or not. The food groups are a good way to ensure a representation of nutrient-rich foods. On packaged foods, you can use the Nutrition Facts panel and the ingredient list to identify nutrient-rich foods and other nutrients you might want to pay attention to, like added sugar, sodium, and saturated fat. You can also look for those nutrients your child may not be getting enough of, such as fiber, or certain micronutrients like calcium, iron, and vitamin D. For example, ready-to-eat cereal falls into the grain food group and is also fortified with iron, zinc, folate, calcium, and vitamin D, making it a good source of nutrients, or highly nutritious. Yogurt, depending on whether it's regular, Greek, or skyr style, has anywhere from 8–15 grams of protein, about 300mg of calcium, plus other nutrients like potassium, phosphorus, and vitamin A. There's a lot of nutrition in a single one-cup serving. Yogurt is a highly nutritious food. If it has some added sugar, it's still decently nutritious, and high amounts of sugar can render it minimally nutritious.

Additionally, certain micronutrients are listed as a percentage of what is needed in the daily diet, stated as a percent Daily Value, or %DV. The %DV helps you determine whether a product contains a

> **#TruthBomb:**
> Knowledge about food and nutrients helps you plan and balance nutritious meals and snacks. Most young children don't need to be bothered with food details, however. The focus for them is to enjoy, learn about, and experience a variety of different foods.

high or low amount of a certain nutrient. For example, 5%DV or lower of iron indicates there's a low amount of iron, while 20%DV or higher indicates it's a high source of iron. The point is to, more often than not, select foods with meaningful nutrients that will benefit your child, and understand that balance and variety are your friends when planning meals and snacks. Overall, it's easier to be flexible and plan nutritious meals and snacks when you look at food through a nutrient lens.

> **#WiseAdvice:** Most of the foods you serve your child in a given day should be highly and decently nutritious foods.

Certain Nutrients Can Increase Satisfaction

Have you noticed that certain foods influence your child's fullness differently? Think about a plate of eggs versus a donut, for instance. What makes eggs more filling and donuts less so boils down to their nutrient content. Studies suggest protein, fiber, and fat can prompt satiety, or the feeling of fullness. The presence of one or a combination of these nutrients in food, a meal, or a snack keeps blood sugar steady and may curtail food cravings. Scientists have even found that two foods with the same number of calories may have different effects on fullness due to their nutrient content.

Protein is the most filling nutrient, followed by fiber, and then fat. When protein-containing foods are eaten they increase thermogenesis, or the amount of energy the body burns after eating. This occurs especially when animal-based proteins such as meat, eggs, or milk are consumed. Body temperature increases and this is interpreted as fullness. A protein-rich meal may also increase the release of gut hormones that cue fullness. Fiber, the source of carbohydrates that most studies focus on when it comes to fullness, is a bit more complex. Fiber can bulk up food, thicken it, or gel in the stomach, with a net effect of feeling full. Fiber-rich foods also distend the stomach, slow digestion, and encourage the release of leptin, signaling fullness. The role of fat in feeling satisfied after eating is less clear. Studies have shown that when people can eat fat without restriction, they overeat. Despite more food consumption, this increase in energy intake does not equal satiety. However, when the diet emphasizes the *combination* of protein, fiber, and fat, satiety awareness improves.

Key Nutrients for Children

Nutrient	What It Does	Consequences of Deficiency
Protein	The building block for normal growth. Needed to build and repair muscles and bones and make hormones and enzymes.	Poor growth, stunted height, higher risk of bone fractures, poor immunity.
Fiber	Helps with normal digestion and elimination. Linked to reduction in heart disease, cancer, and gastrointestinal problems.	Constipation, irregular bowel movements.
Iron	Carries oxygen to organs and cells, helping them function properly. Helps brain development. There are two types of iron: *Heme* is from animals and *nonheme* is from plants. Heme iron is easily absorbed and used; nonheme iron is less bioavailable and needs vitamin C to help the body use it.	Inadequate iron may cause fatigue, paleness, sleep interruptions, and illness. Chronic deficiency causes anemia, which may alter immunity, delay mental development, and lead to poor academic performance.
Zinc	A key nutrient for growth and proper immune functioning.	Poor growth, loss of appetite, lower intellectual capacity, and poor immunity.
Calcium	Makes bones hard and dense with help from vitamin D. Needed for normal muscle contraction and helps blood clot.	Poor bone density; higher risk for osteopenia and osteoporosis; risk for bone fractures; muscle cramps.
Vitamin D	Helps the body absorb calcium. Keeps immune system strong. Plays a role in prevention of chronic diseases.	Rickets, a bone malformation including bowing of the legs or knock-knees. Poor growth and higher risk of fractures.
Omega-3 DHA and Omega-3 EPA	DHA is essential for retina formation and brain development. EPA is needed for blood flow in the brain. Both are essential—humans must get them from food or supplements.	Cognitive delays with deficiency in early life, learning disabilities, vision problems, dry eyes and skin.
Potassium	Helps muscle contract and nerves function; regulates fluid and electrolyte balance.	Fatigue, muscle cramps, and abnormal heart rhythm.

Back to the egg versus the donut: Why is the egg more filling than the donut? It contains protein and fat (egg whites and yolk, respectively). The donut contains sugar and fat. This isn't to say your child should only eat eggs or foods with filling nutrients—donuts are quite enjoyable! Offer donuts occasionally, ideally with a source of filling nutrients, like a glass of milk or a serving of eggs. When you include protein, fiber, and fat in meals and snacks, it will encourage your child's fullness, and this helps *all* kids, no matter their size, better regulate their appetite.

Nutrient Gaps and Deficits

It's hard to believe that nutrient deficiencies exist, especially in a nation where food is abundant. But they do. The most common nutrient deficiencies in *all* children are fiber, potassium, calcium, and vitamin D. Of course, *any* child can be at risk for or have a nutrient deficiency. And although we say children should get their nutrients from food, this can be a lofty goal. For instance, optimal amounts of vitamin D are hard to acquire from food. It's mostly found in fortified milk and eggs, fatty fish, and mushrooms. Although sunshine helps kids activate vitamin D in their skin, we slather on sunscreen, blocking most of this activation. Drinking milk and eating dairy products significantly helps with calcium intake, but kids consume less of these foods after toddlerhood. Getting kids to eat their vegetables has always been a pain point for parents, but the low fiber intake we see in school-age kids comes from a lack of whole grains and fruit, too. And omega-3 fats are found in fish and seafood, items many kids aren't eating. Without enough of these highly nutritious and decently nutritious foods, nutrient gaps may occur. Over time, these gaps can lead to a deficiency or inadequacy, which may affect your child's growth and health, as well as their energy level, sleep, mood, attention, bone development, and immunity.

"Tommy is extremely picky," said Bri, mom to six-year-old Tommy. "He only eats chicken nuggets, pasta with butter, toast, two kinds of cereal, and cheese. I worry whether he's getting enough protein." Picky eaters may eliminate entire groups of food, like fruits, vegetables, whole grains, and proteins, or have a very short list of foods they *will* eat, creating a nutrient gap in their diet. In Tommy's case, he's probably getting enough protein based on his food preferences; however, other micronutrients are in short supply. This is a common scenario in selective eaters—they have a higher deficiency risk for iron and vitamins A, C, and D.

Iron is the most common nutrient deficiency in *all* children, regardless of their size or eating habits, stateside and globally. Iron deficiency and anemia experienced in infancy and in the toddler years are associated with later cognitive disturbances because iron builds the brain structure and its communication pathways. An early iron deficiency may compromise later intelligence. Other nuisances, like constipation, may be due to a lack of fiber in the diet.

Assuming larger and mid-sized children are well-nourished and smaller children are undernourished is a mistake. You can't make an assessment of nutritional status based on a child's size. Furthermore, 20 percent of the children in our nation are food insecure, which means their access to, and ability to afford, nutritious food may be

SHOULD I GIVE MY CHILD A SUPPLEMENT?

If your child is growing well, eating a variety of highly and decently nutritious foods throughout the day, in good health, and doesn't have a documented nutrient deficiency, your child does not need a multivitamin. If your child is selective about food, has an unbalanced diet, or has health challenges like food allergies, a digestive disorder, or another condition that may limit their eating, whether growing well or not, a children's multivitamin may cover questionable gaps in the diet and ease your mind.

If your child has a documented deficiency, like an iron or vitamin D deficiency, they'll need a nutrient supplement to resolve it. For children with larger bodies who have a vitamin D deficiency, supplementation may need to be twice as much (or more) than the dose for children with midsize or smaller bodies. Additionally, studies show the omega-3 index is lower in children with larger bodies; they may need fish-oil supplements, which may also help lower blood pressure, insulin resistance, and triglyceride levels.

unpredictable, interfering with getting enough nutrition. Even financially stable households and highly educated families have nutrient-poor diets. We must look at the whole child and the bigger picture.

Food for Health and Well-Being

For any child with good health and physical functioning, the collective advice is to include highly and decently nutritious foods in the diet, including all the food groups, and place limits on food sources with high amounts of saturated fat, sodium, and sugar. We are learning more about food's influence on health and improving health conditions. From the effects on mood and gut health to adjusting the diet composition to improve health conditions, food can be a tool you can use to your child's advantage.

How Food Helps Mood

Scientists believe mood affects our food choices, but the food we eat also affects our mood. For instance, complex carbohydrates found in foods like sweet potatoes (vegetable group), quinoa (grain group), or rolled oats (grain group) trigger a release of serotonin in the brain. Protein foods, such as beans, tofu, and meats, are linked to increased dopamine and norepinephrine, which play a role in mood, concentration, and motivation. Even fruits and vegetables have been shown to boost happiness. Nutrition research has also identified many nutrients associated with mood, including folate, iron, fats, magnesium, potassium, selenium, thiamine, zinc, and vitamins A, B_6, B_{12}, and C. The bottom line: a variety of foods helps your child's mood and degree of happiness.

How Food Promotes Gut Health

There's a balance of good bacteria and bad bacteria in the gut. Good and bad bacteria both occur naturally in the body, but when we have more good bacteria than bad, we have better gut health. Good bacteria help us digest food, protect against diseases, optimize immunity, improve bowel movements, and more. Probiotics, which are found in foods like yogurt, aged cheeses, kefir, and other fermented foods, like pickles, add healthy bacteria to the gut. Prebiotics are "food" for probiotics and may help boost the growth of good bacteria in the gut. Food sources of prebiotics are fruits and vegetables such as bananas, onions, garlic, and asparagus. Synbiotics are combinations of probiotics and prebiotics, which help probiotics live longer. An example of a synbiotic is the combination of banana and yogurt or asparagus with Parmesan cheese. Good bacteria also communicate with the brain through nerves and hormones, affecting our emotions and how our senses interpret things like smell, flavor, and texture. An unhealthy balance of bacteria (more bad bacteria in the gut than good) may interfere with appetite and confuse hunger and fullness cues.

How Food Improves Health Conditions

It turns out that modifying the nutrient composition of a child's eating pattern may be beneficial for those who have health concerns like hypertension or prediabetes. Food is only supportive, however, and is not "medicine," nor does a single food reverse a medical condition. Let's look at the research about diet composition and how it may improve body function in children with health concerns.

The DASH Diet for High Blood Pressure

The DASH diet, which stands for Dietary Approaches to Stop Hypertension, is rich in fruits, vegetables, low-fat dairy products, and whole grains, and low in processed red meats, sodium, and saturated fats. This plan is low in total fat, saturated fat, and cholesterol and high in the nutrients associated with lowering blood pressure such as calcium, potassium, magnesium, protein, and fiber. The DASH diet is also low in salt. In children ages five to seven, the DASH diet may significantly reduce blood pressure. If your child has high blood pressure, discuss the DASH diet with your health-care provider. The National Heart, Lung, and Blood Institute also offers a comprehensive guide on high blood pressure and how to implement the DASH diet.

The Mediterranean Diet

The Mediterranean diet is characterized by eating vegetables, fruits, nuts, cereals, whole grains, and olive oil; a moderate intake of fish and poultry; and low amounts of sweets, dairy, and red meat. It's rich in monounsaturated fats and fiber, and very low in saturated fat. The

Mediterranean diet has been identified as a prevention diet for health conditions in children, especially if adopted during the preschool years.

A Plant-Based Diet

Cutting down on or eliminating animal foods in favor of more plant foods may improve health. There are a variety of plant-focused diets, including a diet free of all animal foods (vegan), and vegetarian eating patterns such as lacto-vegetarian (consumes dairy products), ovo-vegetarian (eats eggs), and lacto-ovo vegetarian (eats both eggs and dairy). Research shows that a diet that emphasizes fruits, vegetables, nuts, and whole grains, and limits added sugar, refined grains, sweetened beverages, fast food, calorie-dense snacks, and high-fat processed foods, results in a diet lower in calories and fat, and higher in fiber. However, the research in this area has generally focused on adults, and strict plant-based eating patterns may unintentionally miss important nutrients for growth and development in children, especially vitamin B_{12}, iron, calcium, and vitamin D, if they aren't carefully planned.

Other Diet Modifications

If you've heard of certain eating patterns, such as controlling carbohydrate intake (low-carb diet or low–glycemic index diet), low-fat diets, time-restricted eating (intermittent fasting), or a high-protein diet, as helpful for children with health conditions, beware: these eating patterns are generally restrictive and *carry their own set of risks*. They may not be realistic, sustainable, or psychologically safe for children. If you're curious, talk with a health-care provider so that your child's physical *and* emotional well-being is supported.

An Eating Pattern for Better Growth

For children who are not growing well, increasing eating opportunities throughout the day, such as offering three meals and three snacks per day, may help. Boosting calories with added fat and attention to good protein sources can be helpful, too, but remember, these nutrients may induce early fullness. Some families make the mistake of adding too many minimally nutritious foods in this situation. Even if your child is smaller, a highly and decently nutritious diet is the way to go.

Children's current eating patterns have room for improvement, especially in two areas. They should eat more highly nutritious foods, especially fruits and vegetables, and they should consume fewer minimally nutritious foods like sweets and treats. But don't eliminate minimally nutritious foods, as this gives them more power. Remember, it's all about flexibility and balance. Your efforts to instill better food balance now, while your child is young and impressionable, will help them later.

Takeaways:

- Highly and decently nutritious foods should be the anchor of your child's diet, as they provide a good source of nutrients and prevent deficiencies and inadequacies.

- A "nutrient lens" will help you choose highly and decently nutritious foods and balance them in your child's overall eating pattern. Certain nutrients like protein, fiber, and fat help children feel fuller after eating.

- Certain food patterns may optimize health and improve health conditions like high blood pressure.

OBSTACLES AND OBJECTIONS
Minimally Nutritious Foods and Food Shaming

Kids love tasty, appealing foods and they're naturally drawn to sweets. After all, they're bathed in sweet amniotic fluid during pregnancy and some are fed breastmilk early in life, which is naturally sweet. Kids also like attractive, colorful food, and minimally nutritious foods have vivid colors and eye-catching packages. The most obvious obstacles you face as you try to provide your child with an adequately nutritious diet are minimally nutritious foods, portion sizes, and the guilt that comes from food shaming.

Minimally Nutritious Foods

Jamal's nine-year-old son, Michael, is always starving after school. Every afternoon he heads right to the pantry for his daily indulgence of chips, then cookies, and then back for crackers. By the time dinner rolls around, he isn't hungry. "You asked me what my child really eats, and when I think about it, it's a lot of junk food," said Jamal. When I suggested these foods were too accessible, a light bulb went off. "I've completely fallen into the habit of purchasing the foods I know he likes and will eat," he said. "But I don't know how to get out of this rut."

Sweets and treats and snacks . . . my kid loves them and I'm struggling to get out of this rut, too! It's nearly impossible to dodge minimally nutritious food. They're not only easily accessible, but they're also tasty, affordable, and enjoyable. Most kids I've met dig in happily, including my own. That's why it's helpful to have a plan for these foods.

Ultraprocessed Foods

Ultraprocessed foods, such as ready-to-eat and ready-to-heat foods, are made mostly from substances derived from food and additives, and may be high in sugar, sodium, and carbohydrates, and low in fiber, protein, vitamins, and minerals. They're high on convenience, affordability, and flavor. The combination of crunch, mouthfeel, and flavor found in many minimally nutritious foods is what food scientists call the *bliss point*. It makes them highly palatable, memorable, and, well, irresistible. Some children who eat a lot of them may develop a habit of eating them, feeding the pleasure centers of the brain, and kicking off a feedback loop that drives more desire for them. It may seem your child is "addicted" to these foods, but it's the brain and habitual eating of them that are the real culprits.

Experts argue about which foods fall into the ultraprocessed food category. Chips, candy, microwave pizza, and other foods seem obvious, but foods like tofu and soymilk blur the lines. Soymilk is considered ultraprocessed by some, but it is a highly nutritious food with a similar nutritional profile to low-fat cow's milk. Similarly, ready-to-eat cereals may be considered ultraprocessed, but they're fortified with nutrients and are an affordable option. They can nourish kids and close nutrient gaps, especially for families in challenging economic situations. Bottom line: not all ultraprocessed foods are minimally nutritious.

Sweet Foods and Beverages

"Every time I take my child to the grocery store, she begs and begs for Pop-Tarts or muffins," said Jennifer, a mom of two kids under the age of six. "I don't want to go overboard with sweets and sugar, yet I don't want to make them 'forbidden fruit.' She craves sweets, and I don't want to contribute to that, either." Over the years, more and more parents have contacted me about their sweet-obsessed toddler or their sugar-sneaking kid. I'd venture to say sugary food is parents' number one food concern. And this makes sense: children are eating quite a bit of it, diet culture demonizes it, and parents are left in the middle, trying to figure out what to do about it.

The WHO recommends less than 10 percent of the diet be from "free sugar," or sugar that's added to foods like cookies or jelly, or included in food through production (e.g., fruited yogurt, sugary cereal, or chocolate milk). They cap sugar at five to ten teaspoons a day and don't consider the natural sugars from foods like fruit and white milk problematic. The 2020 Dietary Guidelines for Americans agree, suggesting less than 10 percent of the calories consumed in the diet come from "added sugar," and give an okay on natural sugars. Despite these sugar goals, it's getting harder and harder for families to follow them, leading many parents to adopt restrictive practices with sugar, which doesn't help the situation.

> **#TruthBomb:** Sugar intake is higher than recommended for kids today. Toddlers and preschoolers are consuming about twelve teaspoons of sugar daily, while school-age kids are in the ballpark of eighteen teaspoons on average.

Do kids love sweets? Yes. Do they get excited when they can eat them? Probably. Can a child appear to be constantly craving sugar? Of course. Does this equal an addiction? Unlikely. There's no evidence that sugar addiction is a thing in kids. Although the pleasure response in the brain is turned on by highly palatable foods, there are other reasons for desiring sugar, like needing more energy during a growth spurt, physical hunger, or eating to

REDUCED-SUGAR FOODS

When you purchase a product labeled "reduced sugar," it likely contains an artificial sweetener. There are eight non-nutritive sweeteners (sugar substitutes or artificial sweeteners) approved by the FDA for use in our food supply, including saccharine, aspartame, acesulfame-potassium, sucralose, neotame, and advantame; stevia and monk fruit are "generally recognized as safe" (GRAS). These sweeteners are 180 to 20,000 times sweeter than sugar, and it's estimated that 25 percent of children are routinely consuming them. Long-term studies show kids develop a preference for sweeter foods when they consume artificial sweeteners and may experience changes to their gut microbiome.

calm emotions. Carbohydrates, which are highly concentrated in sweet foods, signal energy and quickly satisfy hunger, although not for long. The BLAHS, which you learned about in Pillar Five, influence eating, as does a positive association with eating sweets.

Too many minimally nutritious foods, including sugary foods and drinks, may tip the balance of an adequately nutritious diet to an inadequate place. While children are consuming fewer sodas and fruit drinks these days, children and older kids are drinking more sweetened coffee-, tea-, and milk-based beverages. The warnings and limits about sugar may tempt you to eliminate sweets, but you don't have to (nor do I recommend this). You know forbidding sugar causes its own set of problems. Sweets and other minimally nutritious foods are only problematic when they're consumed in generous amounts or too frequently. All-or-nothing thinking around sweets promotes guilt about eating them and a funky relationship with them. All children can enjoy sweets, and they can be an enjoyable part of your child's eating pattern. Again, the key is to *find balance*, and this may change daily due to what's happening, where you are, and what your child is doing. What is a good balance? If minimally nutritious foods make up more than a quarter of your child's daily eating pattern or are completely absent, both of these extremes seem unhelpful. Balance is where they can be included and enjoyed, and where they aren't a central focus.

Food Portions: A Growing Consideration

Food amounts have scaled up over the years and this fact presents its own challenge. The amount a child eats is called a *portion*. The *serving size*, on the other hand, is a standardized amount of food listed on a food package. The purpose of a serving size is to determine a food's nutrient contribution, such as the nutrients obtained from a tablespoon of nut butter, a cup of milk, or a half cup of cooked pasta. Undoubtedly, serving sizes have grown over recent decades. When I was a kid, forty (or so) years ago, the size of the largest fast-food burger, fries, and soda was the same size as the smallest meal available today. Today, a small popcorn at the movie theater easily meets a serving for two or more people. All-you-can-eat buffets, combo meals, and upgrading your fast-food order to a larger size for a financial incentive are ways portion inflation shows up in children's lives.

You may think that eating a larger portion will satisfy your child and help them down-regulate eating later on. But eating larger portions doesn't necessarily result in fullness, and doesn't always help kids eat less later. Furthermore, larger portions may train children to expect them, needing them to feel full. So it's prudent to offer a reasonable or standard amount of food, something I call a "starter portion," based on the age of your child. For instance, when offering all five food groups at the dinner meal, you might serve your seven-year-old a cup of milk, 2 ounces of protein, ½ cup of vegetables, a cup of fruit, and ½ cup of grains. That's a hearty meal and a full plate!

Using "starter portions" doesn't mean your child can't have more food if they're still hungry (nor does it mean they have to eat everything on the plate), but it allows them to check in with their appetite before taking more. For packaged foods, like pasta, canned beans, or cereal, you can find the recommended serving size itemized on the Nutrition Facts panel. Starter portions and daily servings from each food group are located in the Appendix.

Food Shaming, Must-Haves, and Steer Clears, Oh My!

What is that child eating? Food shaming, or the moral judgment about the quality of food one eats, is another obstacle you may face, especially if your child has a larger or smaller body. Much of the guilt and shame felt about food stems from societal biases and diet culture. If you've ever felt bad about letting your child have an ice-cream cone, or not serving up a salad every day, you know what I mean. Unfortunately, *what* a child eats is another lens through which our society evaluates a child's health and worthiness.

Placing vegetables on a pedestal and calling certain foods "bad" is classic food shaming. *Clean, natural, organic,* and *healthy* are all terms that place a "health halo" on food, implying that something is good for us (or superior to other foods). Terms like *junk, toxic, fortified, canned, prepackaged,* or *guilty pleasure* somehow mean that a food is less than, unhealthy, or undesirable. Our language alone elevates food or tears it down. "Natural" on a peanut butter label draws us in, while the reference to sugar as "evil" repels us and changes our perceptions. We're flooded with food messages that lead to impossible standards and destroy the joy of eating, including for our children. Hence the reason I've chosen to focus on the nutrient quality of food over anything else.

Food shaming doesn't serve your child's growing curiosity about food. In fact, it may short-circuit their exposure to a variety of cultural foods and the opportunity to learn about them. At its worst, food shaming is stigmatizing, making the child who enjoys cultural dishes or minimally nutritious foods, or whose food choices are limited by financial forces, devalue themself. The truth is, food shaming comes from a place of privilege—from the ability to make a choice. Not everyone is privy to that.

As our country grows more diverse, foods from different cultures are more available. And at the same time, children are growing up in homes where the food culture of their ancestors may slowly recede, replaced by peanut butter and jelly sandwiches and chicken nuggets. Families shouldn't have to abdicate their cultural foods just to fit into Western-style eating patterns. In other words, your child should be able to enjoy tikka masala (an Indian dish) or jollof rice (a West African dish) at home or at school without being teased. A rich cultural heritage represented in food is something to be proud of!

I encourage you to teach your child to be accepting and curious about all foods. To be neutral about sweets, treats, cultural foods, and packaged, processed foods. Encourage respect for all foods. The truth is: food is just food. Our bodies need to eat lots of different foods each day. The goal is to help your child be curious about *all* foods and learn that there's no shame in liking what you like. Or in enjoying what you eat. Or in getting by with what you can. Your child—and *every* child, no matter their size—needs to eat. Remember, no single food will make your kid healthy, nor will one food destroy their health. It's about the flexible balance.

Takeaways:

- Minimally nutritious foods are the biggest obstacle to diet quality, but being flexible and planning them into meals and snacks can encourage enjoyment without overindulgence.

- Starter portions can help a child get the nutrients they need while helping them tune in to their appetite.

- Food shaming comes from a place of privilege and may lead children to devalue themselves based on what they enjoy or have available to them.

HOW TO STRIVE AND THRIVE

A Flexible Food Balance

Now, let's get to optimizing food balance flexibly and capitalizing on food enjoyment. Remember, your child's food preferences are developing, taking root from repeated exposure and enjoyment. You can make nutritious foods habit-forming by making them obvious, easy, and attractive. And this is easier to do now than at any other time in your child's life.

Satisfaction, Guaranteed

To work toward a flexible and adequately nutritious diet, you'll want to emphasize highly nutritious and decently nutritious foods as often as possible and work on adding a variety of foods. Use the food groups to plan meals and snacks and the nutrient lens if you're unsure of how a particular food might fit in. Aim to include at least three to four food groups (five if you can!) in each meal and two food groups in each snack. Include the filling nutrients protein, fiber, and fat. Here's a suggested step-by-step approach to ensure fullness and satisfaction after eating:

Step 1: Start with a Protein Food

The "king of satiety," protein can be found in meats such as beef, poultry, and fish; eggs; beans, nuts, and soy; or in dairy foods like milk or yogurt. Select a protein food first when planning main meals.

Step 2: Add Fruits and Veggies for Fiber

Offering both fruits and vegetables at meals not only exposes your child to more nutrients, but fruit takes the pressure off of eating veggies if your child is hesitant. Both of these are great sources of fiber, so they will add a filling factor to the meal. A bowl of grapes or berries and some raw carrot sticks or frozen corn will do the trick.

Step 3: Select Grains for More Fiber

Round out your meal plan with whole grains—they're packed with nutrients and fiber. Select whole grain foods like oat bread or brown rice more often than refined grains like white bread or white rice. You'll be hitting that filling factor again.

Step 4: Where Can You Add Fat?

Fats occur naturally in foods like dairy, fish, or meats. If fat is naturally present in the foods you're making for a meal, you don't need to add more (but you can if you want). However, fat does make the meal more tasty and filling, especially when protein and fiber are also on the plate. If you're adding fat, here are some easy ways to include it: sauté vegetables in olive oil, dress salads with vegetable-based oils, or simply serve higher-fat foods like whole-fat dairy foods.

> **#WiseAdvice:**
> Keep mealtime simple. Use a variety of meal themes throughout the week, such as breakfast for dinner ("brinner"), leftovers (must-go), semi-homemade meals, or throw-together meals. Simple is good enough!

Here are some other meal-planning hacks to create nutritious, filling meals:

- Add at least two colorful foods to each meal and at least one to snacks.
- Cover half the plate with plant-based foods (fruit, vegetables, whole grains, and legumes, for example).
- Divide the plate into four equal sections and fill each section with a protein, grain, fruit, and vegetable food. Add a dairy food (or dairy substitute) on the side, like a glass of milk, or on top, like cheese.
- Serve a combination of highly and decently nutritious foods; add a minimally nutritious food alongside for enjoyment.
- Serve a fruit and/or vegetable at every meal.
- Add a dairy food (milk, yogurt, cheese) or a fortified dairy substitute to every main meal.
- Try to incorporate fish twice weekly to get enough omega-3 fats.
- Don't forget water!

To level-up your meal-planning strategy, rotate different foods within each food group. For example, protein could be tuna fish, egg salad, or lunch meat. When you use food groups as a template for planning meals and snacks, you can rotate different foods within the food groups to boost variety. This chart shows how you can use this leveled-up approach, adjusting it throughout the week.

You can use this same step-by-step approach for snacks; however, you'll be planning for only two or three food groups. Again, the goal is to make a filling snack, which means you want to include at least one food that has a source of protein, fiber, or fat. Filling snacks will keep your child satisfied until the next meal. As an example, a snack could be a small container of yogurt with berries and granola (three food groups), peanut butter on crackers (two food groups), or chocolate chip cookies and milk (minimally nutritious plus highly nutritious foods).

Planning for Lunch Using a Food Group Approach

Food Group	Option 1	Option 2	Option 3	Option 4
Protein	Turkey	Peanut butter	Cubed chicken	Vanilla Greek yogurt
Grain	Oat bran bread	White whole wheat bread	Pasta	Granola
Vegetable	Lettuce, tomato	Carrot sticks	Tomato sauce or diced vegetables	Side salad
Fruit	Grapes	Sliced banana	Applesauce	Mixed frozen berries
Dairy	Cheese	½ cup yogurt	Mozzarella cheese	Included in yogurt
Fat	Avocado or mayonnaise	Included in peanut butter	Olive oil	Walnuts and ranch dressing
Lunch Examples	Turkey and cheese with lettuce, tomato, and avocado on oat bran bread; grapes; water	Peanut butter and sliced banana on white whole wheat bread; carrot sticks; yogurt; water	Cold pasta with cubed chicken, diced vegetables, olive oil, and mozzarella cheese; applesauce; milk	Vanilla Greek yogurt with berries and granola; side salad with ranch dressing; walnuts; water

Here are additional tips for creating satisfying snacks:

- Have a snack out and available on the counter when your child returns from school. Make snack foods obvious, so your child doesn't have to scavenge the kitchen and decide what to eat on their own.

- Cut up fruit and veggies during the week so they are handy, easy to offer, and ready to eat.

- Try a snack platter. Set out a small plate with a variety of highly, decently, and minimally nutritious foods, like cheese, whole grain crackers, chips, nuts, chocolate, and dried fruit.

- Be mindful of starter portions. If you're using a family-style approach to feeding, you can still use an age-appropriate portion when preparing dishes for the table.

- Downsize the plates you use for meals and snacks based on your child's age. Use a salad plate for school-age kids and younger. Preteens and teens can graduate to a dinner plate. Use a saucer for snacks.

Strategically Include Minimally Nutritious Foods

Many families struggle to include minimally nutritious foods while keeping an adequately nutritious food balance. There's no right answer here. But when you have a regular plan for including sweets and treats, they'll become predictable. This also allows you to reinforce their anticipation. For instance, instead of stocking ice cream at home, your policy may be to go out to the local ice-cream parlor. Or if your child asks for cookies in the morning, you can let them know you have them planned for an afternoon snack. The goal is to include minimally nutritious foods, so they are an enjoyable part of your child's eating pattern in a predictable way. Thinking through a plan sends the message that sweets and treats are available (not scarce) and an enjoyable part of life. So how can you keep the balance of minimally nutritious foods in a good place *and* empower your child to make decisions around them?

In my other books, I shared the 90–10 Rule. It's a way to balance minimally nutritious foods and teach your child to make decisions about them as they get older. It goes like this: 90 percent of what your child eats comes from highly and decently nutritious foods and 10 percent comes from minimally nutritious foods (reflecting the current guidelines, and what I refer to as "fun foods"). For most kids, this ends up being one to two minimally nutritious foods in a starter portion, on average, each day. For example, this could be an ice-cream pop after lunch, a mini-sized candy bar (or two, depending on your child's age) or two small cookies at snack time, or a serving of potato chips or french fries along with dinner. Keep the following in mind as you develop your strategy:

Make a Plan: Make room for minimally nutritious foods in your daily and weekly meal plans. Plan for what, when, where, and how many sweets and treats will happen during the week.

> **#WiseAdvice:** You can call minimally nutritious foods "sometimes foods," "fun foods," or any other phrase that resonates. Or don't label them at all! Take care not to use derogatory words that support food shaming.

No Strings Attached: When you include sweets and treats on the menu, they are legit to eat and free from rules and limitations. In other words, use a "no strings attached" policy. Your child doesn't need to earn them. This is especially helpful for kids who've experienced scarcity or tight control around sugary or treat foods.

Add in Highly and Decently Nutritious Foods: Add highly or decently nutritious foods when offering desserts or treats, especially at snack time. For example, cookies with milk, a candy bar with a piece of fruit, or some nuts on top of ice cream. Or serve minimally nutritious foods right alongside the main entrée. For lots of kids, sweets are a powerful temptation, and these strategies can neutralize their power. Of course, there's a place for minimally nutritious foods to be enjoyed all by themselves, too.

Focus on Enjoyment: Encourage your child to eat sweets and treats without distraction, so they're mindful and focused on enjoyment. Encourage your child to enjoy the experience of eating *all* foods.

Food Enjoyment: Embrace Food Experiences

It's heartwarming to watch a child enjoy eating food. It's emotionally protective, enhances health, and can be the gateway to food appreciation, moderation, mindfulness, and self-love. But there are other food experiences that may enhance food enjoyment while building your child's skills, self-esteem, and knowledge.

The Joy of Cooking

As early as possible, let your child have hands-on experiences with food in the kitchen. Your toddler can tear lettuce, stir batter, and crack eggs. School-age children can read recipes, bake with supervision, and assemble their own snacks (from the items you determine for snack time). Many preteens are capable of starting dinner, baking, and cooking independently.

Cooking experiences have been shown to boost skills and confidence, encourage food exploration and trying new foods, and can shape food preferences for nutritious foods. In fact, a review study looked at cooking interventions with children and found that cooking programs had a positive influence on how many vegetables children ate, and increased their preference for them.

Get into the Garden

Digging in the ground and caring for a garden may increase your child's willingness to try new vegetables and to eat more of them. Studies of school gardens show that children develop an increased preference for vegetables and eat more of them when they're able to get their hands dirty. In fact, gardens are more effective at spurring veggie consumption than straight-up nutrition lessons in school. If it works in school, it can work at home or in the community garden, too.

Food Tastings

Sensory education, or teaching children about how food smells, tastes, and appears, can heighten a child's knowledge of food while piquing their curiosity and interest. Studies are ambivalent about whether food tastings have a significant effect on food preferences; however, they're useful in helping children with picky eating overcome food neophobia (fear of new food, a typical characteristic of picky eating). Instead of having new foods always show up on the plate, try a food tasting after school. It's easier to create a pressure-free environment then.

The goal is to create enjoyable food experiences that build your child's knowledge, skills, and self-efficacy. Food should be fun! There are lots of ways to harness adventure, exploration, and enjoyment.

THE WHOLE-CHILD CHECKUP
Food

As you process all you've learned in this chapter, let's pause and assess where you're at. Wherever you find yourself, there may be some work to do. First, are you a Learner, Striver, or Thriver?

The Learner: Where Should I Begin?

Start with the easiest thing: Take note of your child's usual foods and sort them by food group, or by highly, decently, and minimally nutritious foods. Find the missing or neglected food categories and make a list of what you might add. For example, if your child doesn't eat fruit, start to experiment. Try new types or preparations, like grapes, apple slices, applesauce, or raisins. If it's vegetables, add easy-to-prepare vegetables like an iceberg wedge with dressing, frozen corn, or edamame. Work on *adding* highly and decently nutritious foods to the mealtime menu and snack routine. You'll automatically improve the overall nutritional content of the diet.

Next, intentionally incorporate the satiating nutrients. How could you add more fiber? Try mixing whole and refined grains. For instance, take white rice and mix in brown rice, so it's a half-and-half mix. Or purchase white whole wheat bread (it looks the same as white bread) instead of white bread. Mix high-fiber cereal into your child's favorite breakfast cereal. Of course, getting the vegetable and fruit groups on the menu will help bump up fiber, too. What about protein? Plan a protein source at each meal, and consider it at snack time. Go for plant-based fats, like olive oil, nuts and nut butter, seeds, and oily fish and vegetables, like salmon and avocado.

Come up with a plan for how and when to include minimally nutritious foods. Dessert alongside dinner? Savory snacks as part of snack time? A plan will be easier to follow and explain to your child, ultimately cutting down on power struggles and food fights. Find ways to involve your child. Maybe you bake on the weekends or start a summer garden. Or try a food tasting before adding new food to the family meal. Take the path that makes the most sense to you. And if you need help, a registered dietitian is a good place to start.

Food: Learner, Striver, or Thriver

	Learner	Striver	Thriver
Food Fluency, Nutrients, and Health	The daily eating pattern lacks food variety. Large portions are served. A nutrient deficiency exists or is suspected. Erratic presence of satiating nutrients at meals and snacks.	Inconsistent food variety. Protein, fat, and fiber make an appearance, but not routinely. Food portions are a challenge, especially for favorite foods. There are potential nutrient gaps.	Food variety makes nutritional deficiency unlikely. Satiating nutrients are planned into all meals and most snacks. Child is aware of appetite and eats portions that match appetite.
Minimally Nutritious Foods and Food Shaming	Sweets and treats are a significant part of the diet. Family uses "good" food and "bad" food language, potentially setting up food shaming and guilt.	Sweets and treats tend to get out of control when outside the home, but there's a plan for eating them at home. Family realizes food shaming is harmful to child and to others; minimizes polarizing talk about food and eating.	A balance of all foods exists in the home. Understands the nuance around food security, culture, and choices. Allows flexibility with all foods, including minimally nutritious foods. Doesn't polarize food.
Food Enjoyment	Child seems to enjoy only minimally nutritious foods. Parent worries and returns to old feeding habits like restriction. Child lacks hands-on food experiences.	Family is beginning to connect enjoyment to health and well-being. Parent may still emphasize "healthy" food language but is working on food neutrality. Child periodically gets hands-on experiences with food.	Child enjoys all foods. Family knows enjoyment is key to good health and well-being. Child able to cook (with supervision), garden, and have other exploratory experiences with food.

The Striver: Let's Level Up

If you're already food fluent and on the path to food balance, then it's time to level up. Be more strategic with satiating nutrients, for instance. Handling minimally nutritious foods like sweets and treats can be nuanced and challenging. Try a new strategy! Suspect a nutrient deficiency? Get your child checked. And if your child's eating is still a challenge or feels out of control, review Pillars Four and Five, digging deeper into feeding and eating. Drop the food shaming—it shapes a negative food culture in your home.

Give your child more responsibility and freedom in the kitchen. Don't fret if your child only wants to bake. This is normal. Kids start with their familiar, preferred foods, which are often baked goods. They'll move on with time, opportunities, and practice.

The Thriver: Keep Up the Good Work

You've got this. Keep it up, stay aware of food balance, and be flexible. Food needs change as your child ages, so anticipate upticks in appetite, growth, and nutritional needs, especially when puberty is on the horizon. The goal is for your child to learn about food, enjoy it, and meet their nutritional needs with a balance of all foods.

There's no Wi-Fi in the forest,
but you'll find a better connection.

—UNKNOWN

....

....

SCREENS AND MEDIA
The Seduction and Swindle

O ur family moved from one state to another in 2012, and my ten-year-old son spent lots of time playing Minecraft, a three-dimensional video game in which players can build anything. He was a LEGO lover from an early age, and the shift to playing Minecraft was a natural draw. It also filled a void. "Minecraft allowed me to be creative," he said. "I would get up on a Saturday morning, have nothing to do, and start playing. Before I knew it, the day was over." In a way, Minecraft was a saving grace—it occupied my son during a time of chaos and transition. But it quickly got out of hand. Not only was he disappearing into his room for hours, but he was also more and more committed to gaming, which became a barrier to making friends and getting involved in his new community. We had to set some (significant) limits. But we were worried. We knew video games with online friends meant fewer real-life interactions with other kids, but we were wary of restricting access because it took away his primary peer connections. It was a tricky time for all of us (and it was not my proudest parenting moment).

I share this story with you because I know the blessing and curse of screen time for your child. I've experienced the good and the bad. The beautiful moments of family bonding over a Saturday night movie. The distorting Snapchat filters evoking hysterical laughter. The frustrating times when my kids would sit on the couch scrolling on their smartphones when they could be helping me with dinner. And some heart-wrenching cyberbullying on social media.

Whether you like it or not, screen time is part of your reality as a parent. Today, kids are encouraged to hop on the computer as part of their learning. Interactive apps and iPads keep toddlers and preschoolers occupied. Children have phones so we can keep track of them or for use in case of an emergency. There's almost no way around screens and digital media today.

To complicate things further, digital media constantly changes, throwing you new challenges to deal with, from inappropriate content and getting "canceled," to diet culture and rising body image and mental health concerns associated with using them. Those warped Snapchat images might cause damage instead of light-hearted fun. Anxiety-provoking for any parent, yes, and potentially risky for your child. The goal of this chapter is to help you understand the role and risks of media, navigate roadblocks, and help your child engage in ways that protect both their physical health and emotional well-being. Ready?

SCIENCE AND SOCIETY
The Good, Bad, and Ugly

"When Jared was little, I could tell him no more TV and he would get up, turn it off, and happily go play," said Suzanne. "Now that he's older, he gives me all kinds of reasons to keep watching, along with some sass." Unsurprisingly, digital and social media draw kids in. The more they use television, games, and smartphones, the more they want them. Like Suzanne, some parents grow more concerned about the hold digital and social media has on their children, especially how it might shape their attitudes and, more important, the wear and tear on their health behaviors and emotional stamina.

Media isn't a novel worry for parents. My parents worried about how much time my siblings and I spent playing Pong. That was over forty years ago! Twenty years ago, I worried about how much television my kids were watching, the content they were exposed to, and how much time they spent playing video games. During my parenting years, social media platforms emerged. My oldest child begged to have a phone when she was in sixth grade. She wanted a Facebook account, too. My husband and I resisted, but we also felt "parental peer pressure" to allow both. It felt like we were swimming upstream. "I'm the only one without a phone!" cried my daughter. My husband and I sat down and made real decisions about social media and screen time. We came up with parameters, including when my daughter could have access (eighth grade) and the rules of engagement. These guidelines weren't just for her. We were carving out a plan for the next three kids in line.

"At the time, I was so mad I didn't get a Facebook account," said my now-adult daughter. "I'm grateful I wasn't exposed to another outlet for comparison at that age, where people were dressing up their lives on social media. Middle school is tough anyway. I appreciate having the extra years to learn what having an internet presence really means. Now I think eighth grade is too young!" Back then, she wouldn't listen to my concerns about how social media might impact her relationship with her body, or instill more anxiety or even depression. Now she knows.

Digital media has evolved over the years to include many forms. From Atari's Pong in 1975 and the first cell phone in 1983 to the launch of Facebook in 2006 and a slew of other social media platforms, we use media for entertainment and communication. Today, traditional media is supplemented with digital media—a place where any person can consume content and create it. For children, media means a range of applications (apps), multiplayer video games, music, television programming, photographs, videos, and vlogs (video blogs). Information is shared across a variety of these formats. For the purposes of this chapter, I'm zoning in on the digital media that's most influential on children today.

Trends in Digital Media Use

The latest reports indicate kids spend more time engaged with digital media than what is recommended. In toddlers and preschoolers, time in front of screens is roughly two and a half hours per day, and five- to eight-year-olds spend about three hours in front of screens daily. Eight- to twelve-year-old children average six hours of digital media daily overall, with eight-year-olds averaging 4.5 hours per day and twelve-year-olds a whopping 8.25 hours. Shockingly, media exposure begins as early as *four months of age*. Boys play more video games, and girls interact with social media more. A third of the time children spend with digital media involves multitasking, like playing video games while listening to music.

Most parents report their child watches television for more than two hours a day. And over recent decades, more and more kids have access to digital devices such as smartphones, tablets, and computers, shifting how they watch and engage with media. Recently, there's been an explosion in watching online videos over any other media engagement. Specifically, children are watching more YouTube and TikTok videos. Unfortunately, these outlets may lack educational value and may expose kids to violence, advertising, and other age-inappropriate content. With the pandemic, digital media engagement increased even further. Online schooling was necessary and encouraged, producing greater time online for most kids, and reinforcing a habit of physical inactivity.

A survey of parents with children under eleven years gauged the use of screens and social media beginning in March 2020 and again a year later. Nearly across the board, engagement with screens, such as tablets, smartphones, game consoles, or portable gaming devices increased. Another recent survey measured screen time among six- to ten-year-olds and eleven- to seventeen-year-olds, finding that about 33 percent and 39 percent, respectively, had excessive screen time and problematic usage. Higher usage was seen in families with more stressors.

As smartphones have become more available to children, app and social media use have increased. Kids and teens are constantly connected to their digital worlds and some feel "addicted" to their phones. Rather than one social media site, kids have social media "portfolios," where they actively engage on several social media sites. YouTube leads the pack in popularity, with TikTok, Instagram, Snapchat, and Facebook following.

Hours of engagement aside, the impact of media is much more nuanced. Whether media has a positive or negative impact on your child depends on several factors: the type of media being used (TV, computer, video games, etc.); the actual content being watched or engaged with; the context (whether they participate alone or in groups); individual traits (gender, age); and whether they multitask with other media, like playing online games while watching videos. Not all media is bad. As with many things in life, there's a balance to strike. Let's look at what the research has to say about the pros and cons of digital media on children's health and well-being.

The Good News About Screen Time

High-quality media can be engaging, entertaining, and educational for any young child, especially if the child engages with an adult. First, there's nothing wrong with enjoying a show, playing a game, watching a video, or listening to music for the pure enjoyment of doing so. I watched *Mister Rogers' Neighborhood* when I was a kid and allowed my kids daily time in front of the television with their favorite programs. Not only did letting them watch buy me some time to swap out the laundry, but I also felt it was good, entertaining, and educational stuff, reinforcing messages of kindness, caring, and emotional intelligence. Screens can enrich the lives of children when used appropriately. You'll get no guilt trip from me!

Screen time can be of benefit to your child especially when it centers on:

- Face-to-face interactions with family members or friends with whom they cannot physically get together. This is appropriate even for infants and very young children when an adult is present.
- Co-viewing and co-playing with children, especially with video, television, gaming devices, and apps. Asking questions and enjoying play together is a positive experience for kids and helps them have more meaningful interactions.
- Watching high-quality programming. Check out websites such as PBS Kids, Common Sense Media, and Sesame Workshop for their analysis of programs, apps, and more. These will help you make decisions about appropriate content for your child.

- Promoting school readiness, reinforcing school learning at home, and helping your child navigate challenging homework (hello, Khan Academy!).
- Community and creativity for older kids. Social media can be a place where kids can unite on common ground, like the body positivity movement.

Younger children, especially, benefit from interactive media and joint engagement with an adult. They learn better with human interaction, rather than passive, two-dimensional characters on a screen. Studies show that passive learning from an app, video, or program doesn't measure up to real human interaction. For one, the eye gaze isn't directed at the child, and the back-and-forth dynamic of human behavior is lost. Additionally, watching a screen, whether it be TV or a tablet, is sedentary. It's better for young kids to move and engage with the world around them, rather than sit and passively watch. For older kids who engage with social media, building a network of community and a creative outlet are some of the potential benefits.

And Here's the Bad News

You instinctively know there are negative trade-offs with digital media engagement, but do you *really* know what these are? From preteens being at higher risk for eating disorders as a result of pro-anorexia messaging to being "canceled," cyberbullied, exposed to unsavory content, and having their privacy breached, digital media may negatively impact your child's physical and emotional health. Let's explore what might be happening when your child engages with digital media, including their changes in cognitive abilities, interruptions in sleep, reduced daily movement, and mental health concerns. There's a long list of potential negative ramifications tied to screen time.

Behavior. Aggressiveness, distractibility, defiance, and other swings in behavior may show up after your child has spent time playing video games or scrolling social media. School-age children who engage more with media experience an increase in ADHD-like symptoms, such as inattention, impulsivity, and behavioral changes. "Media multitaskers," or kids who use different types of media simultaneously, like surfing the internet while watching TV, have even more symptoms of behavioral change. For instance, heavy media multitaskers perform worse on task switching and tasks that require working memory or focused attention compared to light media multitaskers. They also experience lapses in attention, which is why their performance and behavior suffer. The younger the child, the worse these effects can be, especially on their executive functioning skills. Additionally, being kind to others and other pro-social behaviors plunge as media use increases, while social anxiety and depression rise.

Gaming, specifically, has been studied to better understand the impact on children's behavior and sociability. The more hours of video game play (over nine hours) per week that school-age children engaged in, the more problems with conduct and socially uncooperative behavior they had (kids being less kind to others). But gaming may be beneficial, especially if it's for less than an hour each day, as it may improve social relationships. These studies suggest there's a sweet spot where some video gaming may be of benefit, and too much, detrimental.

Anxiety and Depression. "My daughter is constantly on her phone," said Tessa, the mom of a ten-year-old. "It really scares me, especially when she asks for makeup and other things I think she's too young for." What children do and see in the cyber world, especially as they get older, can be troublesome. On the one hand, social media and gaming can be a way for children to connect, but it can also be a vehicle for destructive behavior and unhealthy comparisons.

Does media use in general increase the risk for anxiety and depression? When toddlers and preschoolers view media for more than four hours a day, they are more unpredictable and dysregulated with their emotions, especially anger. Additionally, more media engagement is correlated with poor conduct, a lack of kindness and caring, and delayed language development and communication abilities. As kids get older, more depression, behavior challenges, emotional concerns, moodiness, anger, and sleeplessness occur. And in the preteen years, high media engagement correlates to depression, anxiety, negative outlook, mood swings, and greater health complaints.

#TruthBomb: As children grow up, engaging with screens is increasingly detrimental to their mental health.

Furthermore, watching videos is linked to depression, and video gaming, texting, and chatting are tied to anxiety. Kids who excessively use electronic media on the weekends may be more inclined toward depression, as they use screens as a way to cope with loneliness and negative emotions. And remember those media multitaskers? They have the highest risk for mental health concerns.

When children have undesirable thoughts, feelings, and other negative experiences, such as being left out of a sleepover on the weekend, ostracized by their peers, or, like my son, being in a new town and not knowing anyone, they want to avoid them. They may engage in what experts call *experiential avoidance*. It's a way to ease these negative sensations, and one reason children are drawn to digital media, particularly if they have anxiety or depression. Ironically, engaging with social media may cause kids to feel more anxious and depressed, especially after using platforms like Facebook, X, Snapchat, or Instagram.

> **#WiseAdvice:** Get your child outside for "green time." Being outside in nature is psychologically favorable for children, reducing their stress and restoring attention. Unfortunately, US kids spend fewer than six hours outside in nature *per week*.

Cognition and Academic Achievement. Video games, especially action-oriented ones, have been associated with improving response time, cognition, and attention control in children. However, when children use more than one media outlet at the same time, they are more distractible, which affects their ability to focus and stay focused. In four- to eighteen-year-olds, watching television or playing video games had the biggest negative impact on academic performance in school compared to any other screen type.

Sleep. Screen use during the day, evening, and in the bedroom may interfere with your child getting a good night's sleep. During the day, frequent use of screens, highly interactive content, and violent content delay the onset of sleep and may interrupt the quality of zzzz's your child gets. At night, especially the hour before bedtime, watching TV, playing a video game, or scrolling social media impairs the quality and duration of sleep. And it's almost a guarantee that your child will shorten their sleep time, quality, and efficiency if they have screens in the bedroom, especially if they're using a mobile device in a dark room, or have multiple screens there (television, computer, and smartphone, for instance).

Body Size. For the most part, screen time is sedentary. Studies have tied too much screen time to eating more food and choosing sugary, higher-fat, and calorie-rich foods. Efforts at reducing screen time, while helpful in many areas, do not change a child's size or health concerns.

Screen Time Recommendations for Children

Age	Recommendation	Appropriate Use
2 to 5 years	< 1 hour per day	Co-view and co-play with an adult.
5+ years	At parental discretion	Put in place a media-use plan, screen time limits, and age-appropriate content.

Screens are like a "frenemy"—they offer positive enhancements to your child's life, but they can also be a bad influence. It's easy to pinpoint screen time as something to modify, but it's hard to separate it from physical activity, food choices, eating habits, and sleep when it comes to overall health. You can use screen time to your child's advantage while staying aware of how it may influence and impact your child's health and well-being. If it feels like your child is getting too much screen time, they probably are.

Takeaways:

- Children engage with screens as young as four months of age and most exceed viewing and engagement recommendations.
- For children two to five years, less than an hour a day is recommended. For kids older than five years, parental discretion and limits are advised.
- Screen time may enhance education and executive function, and sustain connections with others, but too much can have negative repercussions on kids' health, well-being, and behavior.

OBSTACLES AND OBJECTIONS
From Cyberbullies to Food Marketing

According to a recent survey, 66 percent of parents believe parenting is harder due to technology and social media. Online privacy concerns, cyberbullies, and exposure to eating disorder tips are top worries. Let's dive into what sets children up for being highly engaged screen users, as well as some of the insidious risks inherent to screens, like thin idealism and diet culture, food marketing, and cyberbullying.

The Models of Media

Parents who have the habit of using screens set an example for their children. High parental screen use, such as television viewing, surfing the internet, playing games on a smartphone, or liking, commenting, and engaging with social media channels, shows your child when and how to engage. Parents with high screen use, especially mothers, have children with higher screen use. How mothers interact with screens, using them as a distraction at mealtime, or employing them to control a child's behavior either as a form of discipline or a bribe for better behavior, are some of the leading contributors to a child's engagement with screens. Fathers who use screens at mealtime influence their children's screen use as well.

Parental self-efficacy is the belief that you're a good parent, and you can shepherd your child to good habits. High parental self-efficacy is associated with confidence in learning and practicing effective parenting skills. On the flip side, parents with low self-efficacy have a hard time navigating challenging parenting situations, like a child who is heavily engaged with screens. Parental self-efficacy is key to having a positive influence on your child's development, habits, and health. Parents who have confidence in their parenting skills, especially around regulating screen use, have children who engage *less* with screens and who fall within screen time recommendations. In other words, if you think you can successfully manage your child's screen time, you can.

#TruthBomb: More than half of parents (56 percent) say they spend too much time on their smartphones, 36 percent say they spend too much time on social media, and 11 percent say they spend too much time playing video games.

Household Chaos

We are late to everything. I cannot hear myself think, it's so loud. Where's your coat?! Household chaos means there are higher levels of confusion, disorganization, and hurriedness in your home. We all have this occasionally, but if it's the norm, it can affect your attention and stress levels, and your parenting abilities. One study found that chaotic households, independent of household characteristics (socio-economic status, education, race, etc.), had preschoolers with high screen usage, using them an hour before bedtime, and having them in the bedroom. Because screen engagement starts early in life, and increases as children age, developing calm routines, rules, and a strong set of parenting skills will help you and your child develop good habits around screen time.

Social Media: A Hotbed of Diet Culture and Thin Idealism

The incidence of eating disorders increased during the pandemic, and studies show that hospital admissions for eating disorders during this time, when screen time and social media engagement were at an all-time high, increased by 48 percent. In a *Wall Street Journal* article entitled "'The Corpse Bride Diet': How TikTok Inundates Teens with Eating-Disorder Videos," author Tawnell D. Hobbs writes about how the platform's algorithm can take teen viewers down a rabbit hole of emaciated individuals, body-shaming, and dangerous dieting techniques. And it keeps feeding this stuff to them. Furthermore, in 2021, Facebook, TikTok, and Instagram faced concerned senators in a hearing over the content of their respective platforms and how each may be promoting subject matter that triggers, contributes to, and glamorizes eating disorders.

#TruthBomb: Kids as young as eight years use social media, and usage increased by 17 percent between 2019 and 2021.

Social media platforms are part of diet culture—idolizing thin bodies and the means by which thinness is attained and sustained while stigmatizing larger bodies and supporting biased beliefs against them. These platforms offer a place where children and preteens can shame, or be shamed. Where they can learn and be inspired, for better or worse. Where they'll likely compare themselves to others.

Your thirteen-year-old may be comparing themself to a twenty-four-year-old who's used filters, plastic surgery, or protein supplements to create a perfect image. Unable to identify what's real and what's not, and because they're strangers, it's easy for your child to assume everything is natural. They'll notice the thousands of likes and comments, and witness others applaud this individual based on their looks, which will increase their desire to look like them. Children and preteens are especially impressionable, and social media content can sway their thinking and decision-making to dangerous and unhealthy behaviors.

Social media may contribute to body image concerns and emotional distress by promoting "healthy" foods, thin bodies, unfounded nutrition advice, weight loss, and exercise. Platforms that do this receive high levels of engagement, especially among young people. Youth who are engaged with digital photo–based platforms seem to be especially affected. In middle school students, the influence of image-oriented social media on a child's awareness, sense of pressure, and internalization of body ideals predicted body image and eating problems. Specifically, social media usage *significantly predicted* whether a child was concerned about their eating, body weight, and shape, and whether they restricted their eating. Both boys and girls are affected—boys more so

THE SOCIAL MEDIA ALGORITHM

An algorithm is a set of rules and signals that sends social media users toward content they are iikely to engage with. For instance, if your child likes, clicks, or comments on posts about baking, they'll see more posts about baking. The algorithm learns, based on your child's interactions and behavior, what they like and what they want to see. You can see how hard it can be for them to get off media when the content they're likely to engage with keeps showing up. Also, because it's based on their behavior, social media's algorithm creates a self-fulfilling feed, or echo chamber—showing them what they like—instead of other opinions, topics, or alternative activities.

Some companies have been called out for creating algorithms that show increasingly more upsetting or unsuitable content to children. For example, if your child likes animals, they may start to see content that shows animal cruelty. Or if your child watches fitness videos, they may eventually see content that extolls extreme exercise or unhealthy weight loss behaviors. The algorithm can also push food advertising, targeting children based on their online behavior. It can also point your child to body-positive accounts, which is a good thing, but you have to train it to do so.

#WiseAdvice: You should feel empowered to keep track of your child's activity and connections on social media. Monitor their feed, and block, unfollow, or report any inappropriate content.

by *awareness*, which predicts more concerns about eating, and girls by *pressure*, which incurs more concerns about eating, weight, and shape.

Cyberbullying: What They Say Does Matter

Cyberbullying is bullying online. It's mostly characterized by spreading rumors, name-calling, and sharing pictures or videos on social media platforms. More problematic than face-to-face bullying, cyberbullies can strike hard and fast, and spread their messages widely. "What's so different today for kids who are being teased and bullied, is that it just never gets turned off, because of social media," said Dr. Rebecca Puhl, deputy director of the University of Connecticut Rudd Center for Food Policy and Health. "Having that 24/7 kind of access to disparaging comments and shame is so debilitating emotionally." Twenty-three percent of middle and high schoolers have experienced cyberbullying, and this is strongly associated with depression. Victims of cyberbullying are also at higher risk for self-harm and suicidal behaviors.

Children with larger bodies are targets for all types of bullying and victimization, but especially cyberbullying, which can contribute to poor self-esteem and a greater likelihood of gaining body fat in the future. Children who are larger are likely to experience anxiety and depression as a result of any type of bullying (physical, cyber-, verbal, etc.), and children in very large bodies internalize these symptoms to a greater degree than their peers of any other size. Furthermore, boys, rather than girls, with *smaller* bodies or who are underweight, experience greater body dissatisfaction as a result of bullying.

Kids with larger bodies tend to deal with bullies by using avoidance as a coping skill. One study found almost 90 percent of teens with larger bodies experienced bullying related to their size. Fifty-three percent said they stood up for themselves, tried to educate their bully, helped others who were being bullied, or became a bully themselves. Ninety-four percent said they faked indifference, denied it was happening to them, isolated themselves, or self-harmed. Almost half used a combination of both coping strategies. But here's the kicker: *almost all* kids in larger bodies are bullied and *almost all* of them use avoidance to cope. Avoidance is a negative coping skill and is associated with adverse mental health symptoms, low self-esteem, and negative body image. Although this study showcased teens, it adds an important futuristic lens for parents of younger kids and preteens.

> **#WiseAdvice:** Support and help children of all sizes be good humans. Kids with larger and smaller bodies are targets of bullying, especially cyberbullying, and may need more emotional support.

Food Marketing: I See It, I Like It, I Want It

The Rudd Center for Food Policy and Health at the University of Connecticut is a hub for research about food marketing to children.

Food is primarily advertised to kids via screens—television, smartphones, tablets, and computers. Television is the main source of marketing to children, and advertisers spend close to $11 billion advertising food and beverages to them. As TV viewing has decreased with the rise of social media engagement, food marketers are following the trend, placing food and drink ads and messaging on social media platforms, branding games, and using "ambassadors" to promote their products. Often, food marketing is disguised as entertainment, capitalizing on the natural appeal to children.

Children of color are targeted with food advertising more than white children. What's worse? The ad content they see is for minimally nutritious foods, like candy, fast food, and sugary drinks, contributing to the greater health concerns we see in communities of color. Although there's been a major downshift in television advertising to children between 2017 and 2021, there's also been more spending on advertising for unhealthy food products on social platforms targeting Black and Hispanic youth, even when food companies have more nutritious products they could be advertising to them.

What does food marketing do to your child? It shifts their food preferences to the foods that are being advertised to them. Kids increasingly desire these foods, ask their parents for them, and consume more of them. Fast food is the most aggressive category of food marketing to children, and sugary beverages like soda, sports drinks, and fruit drinks follow. Misleading nutrition claims on the front of food packages like "30% reduced sugar" or "all-natural ingredients" can sway parents to believe sugary foods, beverages, and fast food are good for their kids. Children who see ads for food pester their parents to buy those foods. Do not be fooled, my friend. This is marketing strategy at its best: altering your beliefs through confusing and misleading nutrition information while capturing your child's interest so they influence your decisions.

Now that you understand the good, bad, and dark sides of digital media, let's explore how you can help your child be a good steward of screen time and keep it in its proper place.

························· **Takeaways:** ·························

- How digital media is handled in your home influences the screen time habits your child develops.

- Social media perpetuates a focus on appearance and may be a source of stigma, challenging your child's body image and self-esteem.

- Food marketing targets children and influences food attitudes, preferences, and purchasing decisions.

HOW TO STRIVE AND THRIVE
A Safe Media Diet

Although you may want to just eliminate screen time altogether, it's not practical in today's world. Your child will likely be introduced to screens at a young age and the exposure will naturally ramp up. So how can you approach screen time in a way that encourages your child to reap the benefits and downplay the dark side?

Calm the Chaos at Home

"I couldn't get anything done when Taylor was younger unless I parked him in front of a video," said Tracy. "Now, I can't drag him away!" For many parents, screens have become a way to cope with busyness and stress, and a way to distract and entertain kids. If you find yourself using the television or iPad to babysit your preschooler or child, or are relieved that your preteen squirreled off to the bedroom to play a video game alone, there may be too much chaos in your home. Chaos leads to more stress. More stress leads parents and kids to look for ways to cope. Screens, as you've learned, are a prime coping tool for kids, and can be a crutch for parents.

To minimize chaos in your home, the obvious answer is to create more order. Systems, routines, and a rhythm to the day become known, expected, and predictable. This doesn't mean that screen time can't be a part of the daily routine. It can. When it's scheduled and predictable, and you're calm about it, you and your child will be less inclined to turn to screens inappropriately. Here are a few ways you can build in more calmness.

Routines and responsibilities. I love routines! From family meals to regular bedtimes, having a framework of activities throughout the day keeps things predictable for your child. Give your child chores and responsibilities like contributing to the family meal, caring for a pet, making their bed, or gathering the laundry. Chores help you out, but more important, they keep kids busy, build their autonomy, and minimize downtime when screens become even more appealing.

Have a designated time for using screens. Maybe your family watches a television program together after dinner, or "video game time" is allowed after homework is completed. For older kids, setting aside a time when they can dive into their social media connections will help them feel like they're getting exclusive time.

Avoid overprogramming. Easy to say. Hard to do. Truth is, many kids are overscheduled. They go to school, an after-school activity or two, and their weekends are full of obligations. While it's good to keep kids busy, it may also keep you in "chaotic mode," with your child seeking ways to unwind. You are the best judge of whether your child's extracurriculars are contributing to the household chaos. To keep things relaxed, consider building in screen-free time, like using the car ride to and from activities to talk with your child rather than using the phone. Screen-free downtime promotes other things that benefit kids' well-being, like getting out in nature, reading a book, talking with an adult, or creating artwork.

Schedule quiet time. When my kids were little, I had "lay me down" time each day after lunch. They went to their rooms, where they could quietly play with their toys, read a book, or write—on their bed. This was quiet, alone time. No screens. Often they rested or took a nap. And I got uninterrupted chore time. Encourage your older child to seek out quiet, screen-free time (reading, journaling, meditating, or stretching, for instance) and showcase it as a way to care for their body and mind. You'll learn more about self-care in the next Pillar.

Daily downloads. As you've learned throughout this book, stress encourages negative coping skills. To combat stress, make sure your child has opportunities for a "daily download." Talking and communicating thoughts, feelings, and events of the day from an early age helps your child open up later when they're older and things get tough. The child who is talking about their day at preschool becomes the child who can tell their parents when they've been bullied or they see something inappropriate online.

Establish the Rules of Engagement

The American Academy of Pediatrics (AAP) advises parents develop a family media plan, noting that negotiating a plan for, and with, the whole family is your best edge for curtailing inappropriate content and too much time on screens. Discuss this plan, answer your child's questions, and role-play scenarios of appropriate and inappropriate use of digital media. The goal is to communicate your expectations and have your child buy into the plan. The following are things to consider as you detail your family's media plan:

Appropriate Content. Decide what is appropriate for your child to view, no matter what type of screen. Remember, just because an app says it's for a certain age group or that it's educational doesn't necessarily mean it is. Head to Common Sense Media or other resources to evaluate games, videos, and programs before allowing your child to view them. For preschoolers, the best apps and games are ones that focus on engagement, like swiping, and those in which your child, not the app, chooses the next step.

Co-viewing and Co-playing. Watch, play, and connect with your child across all media outlets. Engage with your preschooler on interactive programs and apps, co-play video games with your child, and watch movies and videos together. Befriend your older child on social media platforms and monitor the content they're seeing. Specify acceptable use in your media plan, such as video chatting with friends and family, playing learning apps, watching age-appropriate shows and movies, and using media for creative endeavors. Also, delineate unacceptable behavior like going to a new website or social media platform, or watching videos without asking permission first.

Screen-Free Time. Be clear about when screen time is not allowed, such as during homework time, the hour before bedtime, while crossing the street, during family time, meals, dining out, and while in the car. Plan for screen time during the day, but balance it with sleep, physical activity, meals, homework, and school. When you map it out, you may find there's naturally a limited amount of time for screens.

Screen Curfew. Decide when screens are turned off for the day and where they will recharge. Perhaps it will be in your bedroom (not your child's!), a den, or another central part of your home. I recommend you designate a charging hub for all devices.

Screen-Free Zones. Your child's bedroom should be a screen-free zone. No television, computer, or other devices. For older children who may be using computers as part of their schoolwork, consider a laptop rather than a desktop as this can be easily removed from the bedroom at night. Other screen-free zones to consider are the kitchen and the meal table, as screen use here can lead to mindless eating and interrupt the family connection.

Raise a Media Ace

"We have been teaching our kids about media for a long time," said Rob, a PR and media expert. "I know my kids need to understand what the underlying messages are so it doesn't harm them." Media literacy, or the ability to assess and analyze media messages at a deeper level and distinguish their intent and truthfulness, can help your child sift through advertising, marketing, and bias. From fact-checking to a "gut check," media literacy can help them identify credible information, differentiate fact from fake news, and see through ulterior motives.

Deciphering media and its intent helps your child become a critical thinker who recognizes a point of view (and develops their own along the way). Media literacy facilitates savvy consumerism, not simply taking information at face value, but digging in to find the truth. And perhaps most important, it helps your child create their own media responsibly, potentially breaking negative norms of bias and stigma.

Asking Questions. Young children are limited in their cognitive understanding, as you've learned. One way to introduce what's going on behind the scenes on any media platform is to ask the question, *Who is telling the story?* A preschooler might define the storyteller as the main character in an ad, like a mom or child. Naturally, they cannot see the true narrator or the writer behind the ad. But that's not the point. The point is to focus on the storyteller. This lays the foundation for questioning what they view. As children mature, they'll be able to see it's not the mom in the ad: a school-age child can identify an actor telling a story; an older child will know the copywriter is telling one. Your job isn't to get your child to mature faster. Rather, it's to get them into the *habit of asking questions*.

You can also do this with active reading. Rather than reading the words, you ask questions instead. *What color is the unicorn? What will the unicorn do next?* By asking anticipatory questions, you're training your child's brain to assess and make sense of what they see. Again, this is fundamental to becoming a critical thinker. And this becomes a crucial skill when digital media is a bigger part of their lives. Ask older kids, *Why did they create this ad? What are they trying to sell? Why? Is this fact or sensationalism? Does this make sense?*

Another way to help your child understand various forms of media is to have them retell what they see as a story. This enhances comprehension and assessment skills and prepares your child to be a storyteller down the road, which will impact how they create future media.

Lateral Reading. Lateral reading is reading two different stories, articles, or reports side by side and comparing them to corroborate the information. It's a way to fact-check and get to the truth, especially as social media uses splashy headlines to get your child or preteen to click (called clickbait). Unfortunately, children and preteens are vulnerable to clickbait because, developmentally, they believe what they see and hear. Encourage your child to be curious. Sensationalized information exists everywhere—in advertising, social media, and the news. Rather than ingesting this information without question, teach your child to dive in for the truth and to fact-check.

Mike Caulfield, a digital literacy expert, has developed SIFT, an acronym that stands for Stop, Investigate, Find, and Trace, to break down digital messages.

Stop.

Do you know the source of the information? Consider what you already know and why you're seeking this information.

Investigate the source.

Check out the information provider. Can you find them on Wikipedia or a trusted website? Are they the real deal? Some sources promote a particular agenda or viewpoint, rather than the truth.

Find trusted coverage.

Look for the most authoritative information on a topic, which will require a bit of research. Open a new tab to "lateral read" other information. Compile a consensus from multiple sources.

Trace claims, quotes, and media to the original context.

Go back to the original source, whether it be a research paper or a report. Verify the context and actual reporting. Does it match the original source?

Enforce Media Safety

Ensuring your child's safety in the digital world is an active practice. Unfortunately, cyberbullies, online predators who exploit children, and inappropriate content, such as vulgar language or violent or sexual images, are leading threats here. A media use plan helps quite a bit, but you can take additional steps to keep your child safe when they're online.

Make sure websites are secure. Secure websites have a URL that starts with "https." The "s" on the end identifies that the website itself is taking security measures. If it's not there, stay away.

Do not share personal information. If possible, use other login information for your child instead of their name or other personal identifiers like address, phone number, social security number, birth date, or photograph.

> **#TruthBomb:** More than 55 percent of preteens (aged ten to twelve years) have been exposed to violent content and nearly 60 percent have seen (or heard) sexually explicit content.

Delay social media platforms as long as possible. Children and preteens are developmentally sensitive to what they see on social media. The longer they wait to use social media, the more mature and media savvy they'll be. Most experts advise waiting until your child is thirteen years old, or in the eighth grade. If your child does have access to social media, connect there and demand oversight.

Use parental controls. Many of your child's devices, such as Apple and Google products, already have parental controls built in. You'll also find them available on Amazon, Netflix, YouTube, and social media sites. SafeWise, a website focused on safety and security products, reviews parental control apps (some of which are free), so you can monitor your child's activities.

Update, update, update. Make sure your child's devices and software are up to date. Updates are often security-oriented, targeting the latest threats.

Beware of stranger danger. Contact from a stranger online is never okay. Chat rooms and video games are common places where predators show up, often posing as children themselves. Talk about this with your child and discourage any conversation with strangers on the internet. Also, deter your child from clicking on links from someone they don't know, sharing photos with strangers, or agreeing to meet someone they've met online.

> ## RESOURCES FOR MEDIA LITERACY AND SAFETY
>
> *Common Sense Media*: Media reviews and how-to discussion guides on media for parents.
>
> *Critical Media Project*: Activities and videos for kids and parents on identity and representation in the media.
>
> *Informable*: Game-style approach to teaching media literacy on the go.
>
> *MediaWise Teen Fact-Checking Network*: Fact-checks for teens, by teens.
>
> *News-O-Matic*: News app for six- to fourteen-year-olds.
>
> *SafeWise*: Security resources for media use.

THE WHOLE-CHILD CHECKUP
Screen-Time

Now that you know about digital media and screen time, let's see where you're at. How are you keeping screen time in check, and where might you improve in this area? Are you a Learner, Striver, or Thriver? Let's find out.

The Learner: Where Do I Begin?

First, let's tackle the low-hanging fruit: get the screens out of your child's bedroom. Take them off the meal table, too. Find a place where screens can live—in the family room, living room, den, basement—wherever there's a space your child can engage safely with media. A spot where you can easily engage *with* your child and monitor them if they're engaging alone.

Next, create your family media use plan. You can use the AAP's online family media plan (located at https://www.healthychildren.org/english/fmp/pages/mediaplan.aspx) or create one yourself using the parameters outlined here. It doesn't have to be fancy, but I do recommend you keep it

Screens and Media: Learner, Striver, or Thriver

	Learner	Striver	Thriver
Calm Home	Parent is stressed and overwhelmed. The home feels rushed, disorderly, and last-minute. Screens are used as entertainment and distraction so the parent can get things done. Unplanned time and erratic schedules lead to heavy use of screens.	Parent schedules formal time for media. Child has chores, responsibilities, and time in the day for quiet time. Parent gets pushback from the child but understands this is part of the process.	Parent has a predictable flow to the day and child has daily chores, activities, and quiet time built in. There is a balance of activities, including a set time for screens. The home is calm.
Family Media Plan	The family has no formalized media plan in place. Child engages excessively with screens. Child can easily access screens when desired. Screens are in the bedroom.	Family has some parameters for screen use, but they waver between just enough and too much, especially on rainy days or days off from school. Screen-free times and zones are emerging; screens are out of the bedroom. Child will gladly exceed the media plan if parents are distracted.	Family executes a media plan. Screen-free zones and a screen curfew are enforced without complaint. Parent trusts child to respect the media plan and child comes to parent to discuss exemptions.
Media Literacy	Parent has awareness of advertising, clickbait, or agenda-driven news, making it hard to teach the child. Few parental controls or safety rules are in place. Child may be exposed to inappropriate content. Privacy may be compromised.	Parent discusses media intent regularly with child. Child questions the content they're viewing. Some safety controls are in place. Child is learning lateral reading and SIFT.	Family converses about advertising, news, and social media regularly. Child can fact-check information. A media plan, parental controls, and safety rules are in place. Parent regularly updates media sites and programs for optimal security.

flexible. It will change as your child gets older, so it's not a one-and-done thing. Post it centrally for all to see and revisit it to make tweaks.

If you have a young child, you'll have more control of the family media plan, but older kids will need to be included in its creation. Get their input, use their ideas (if reasonable), and make this truly a "family plan." Parents follow the plan, at least during the day, too. Remember to walk the talk. Accountability will be higher if everyone plays by the rules.

Tighten up security. Do the basics like ensuring your computers, smartphones, and subscriptions are up to date with the latest versions. Join your child as they use media and take the opportunity to begin asking questions to critically review the media your child is viewing, be it books and television programming in the case of younger kids, or ads, news, and social media content with older children. Questions are the easiest way to get the ball rolling.

- *I'm curious, what do you think will happen to [character] when [event, activity] happens?*
- *What is the story here? Can you tell it to me in your own words?*
- *How do you think [a friend, your grandmother, your teacher, etc.] would feel if they read or saw this?*
- *What is true about this situation? What do you know to be false?*
- *What do you need to know more about in order to understand this better?*

You don't have to have the answers! It's an exercise in media literacy to go into the digital world and seek the answers. Together, hunt for the truth using SIFT. Remember, teach your child to ask questions and find answers, no matter their age.

The Striver: Let's Level Up

You have rules about screen time in place. Your child knows the rules and seems to follow them. You're feeling pretty good about where screen time fits in your family life, but rainy days, school breaks, and weekends upset the routine. That happens with a lot of families. Downtime often equals more screen time. The antidote to unplanned downtime is to make a plan. I suggest you create a list of activities your child can do alone or you can do together, such as specific nature walks, hikes, festivals, beaches, baking, crafting, and other activities. When unplanned time comes up, you'll have a go-to list of ideas. Even better, ask your child to add to the list, consult it, and choose activities.

Stretch your media literacy by going deeper. Point out size discrimination, stigma, and bias in the media. Negative portrayals of children in larger bodies exist. In the movies, verbal insults about body size normalize this behavior for impressionable minds who are watching. Social media commonly shows aggressive messaging and negative comments toward individuals in larger bodies. Even health-promoting media campaigns can be stigmatizing, especially when they use stigmatizing photos of children with larger bodies. No matter the size or age of your child, you can teach them to spot stigma on social media and in movies, whether it be the thin ideal, lack of body diversity, or negative representation of children and adults of larger or smaller sizes. Plant the seeds of advocacy by first helping your child recognize disparities in the digital world.

The Thriver: Keep Up the Good Work

You're doing great, but your job isn't over. Digital media is quickly evolving and you will have to keep up with the changes. As your child grows up, their interests and the presence of digital media in their lives will likely expand. When employed effectively, media can help your child learn, explore, create, and advocate. But it may also cause harm to your child's mental health and safety when it's not. Stay on top of it!

To be yourself in a world that is constantly trying to make you something else is the greatest accomplishment.

— UNKNOWN

SELF-LOVE
An Advocate for Self

I s it possible to raise a child who likes themselves, let alone *loves* themself? A little person that enjoys *who* they are? *Appreciates* their body? Sees their differences as an asset? As a mom of four, three of whom are girls, I worried that my kids would grow up not liking themselves. It's a weird thought, I know. But in my fifty-plus years, I've encountered too many folks who don't seem to accept themselves. How do I know? I hear them saying things like, *I should've taken better care of my skin. I wish I appreciated my body when I was younger. I need to go on a diet when the New Year rolls around (she says every year since she had babies). I wish I was . . . I'm not [insert shortcoming, perceived failure, or inadequacy].* Of course, we all have those moments, when we rue what could have been. Society has a standard, and it plays into how we feel about ourselves. And if we look outside for confirmation of our worthiness, it's easy to feel "less than." Self-love is the complete opposite. It means we look inside for the standard. It means we know we're good. *We're worthy as is.*

Few people talk about raising a child who loves themself, but I think this is critical to raising *any* child who is confident, resilient, self-compassionate, enough, joyful, and self-advocating. But how do you do it? First, as I covered in Pillar One, it boils down to knowing and accepting the child you have, unconditionally. Second, being seen, heard, and known are the seeds that plant worthiness, confidence, and self-respect. I believe a focus on cultivating self-love is a priority for *every* family raising *every* child, now more than ever.

SCIENCE AND SOCIETY
It's All About the Self

I t's essential for children to figure out who they are and appreciate themselves, and this happens throughout the social and emotional developmental stages of childhood. Riding alongside, however, are the messages and societal norms of today. These norms, which we've talked about throughout this book, may undermine your child's developing sense of self, regardless of their body size, but especially if they have a smaller or larger body. You must counteract these norms with your words and actions, centered on respect, enoughness, compassion, care, and empowerment. These are the seeds that grow into self-love.

Not too long ago, self-love was associated with narcissism, ego, and being selfish. Today, self-love has shifted to a more positive, empowering meaning. Self-love is having a high regard for your own well-being and happiness, and taking care of your needs rather than sacrificing them for others. Psychologists say the more actions your child takes to support their physical, psychological, and emotional growth, the more appreciation they'll have for themself. In other words, they'll be more likely to rate themself highly and have more positive personality traits and behaviors. This self-positivity bias contributes to better mental health, self-acceptance, self-esteem, motivation, determination, and self-awareness.

> **#TruthBomb:**
> Researchers have found that about 50 percent of a child's self-esteem is genetic, and the other 50 percent is informed by the environment they grow up in.

When I was in college, I remember looking in the mirror one day and realizing that I liked myself. Corny as it seems, I said out loud, *"I like you, Jill."* Although I didn't have everything I wanted, didn't *love* every aspect of myself, nor had I achieved all I desired, I had a strong sense that I was good. I was enough. Despite the fact that my parents were divorcing, I felt happy and content with myself at that point in my life. I intuitively knew I had the internal resources to make it.

Of course, I didn't just wake up and decide I liked myself. Back in the eighties, the idea of self-love wasn't really a thing, so it wasn't overtly cultivated in my growing-up years. Liking myself came from years of feedback and love from my parents, family, and friends. From teachers, coaches, and other adults in my life. From the social and environmental privileges into which I was born. From respect, achievement, decision-making, self-direction, self-awareness, and a sense I deserved a place in this world. I had resilience in my back pocket.

Cultivating self-love in children is more than telling your child over and over that you love them. That doesn't necessarily translate to loving themselves. Psychologists say that self-love is built from self-value, self-esteem, self-care, and self-awareness. Let's review how these work together.

> **#TruthBomb:**
> Generation Z, people born between the mid- to late-1990s and the early 2010s, have the lowest ratings of self-love, according to a 2020 survey.

Self-Value: I Exist

Self-value is the belief that you are worthy, simply because you exist. A sense of self-worth means you believe with unshakable confidence that you are valuable. But we humans struggle to believe in ourselves. We tend to focus on the negative: the failings, inadequacies, and not-good-enoughs. We project this negativity onto ourselves and others without even knowing it. For example, a child develops shame about their desire to eat sweets after they're told that these foods are "unhealthy" and "toxic." Or they don't enjoy exercise, but when they hear comments like "lazy," a self-fulfilling prophecy may unfold. And, if *you* struggle with health behaviors, it might be easier to blame yourself or your child for having health concerns rather than address the constraints on your life that interfere with access to food, health care, or a decent wage.

When I was a younger parent, I read or heard somewhere that the simple act of smiling with delight when a child enters the room is a powerful gesture in conveying acceptance and love. Instead, so many of us (myself included) greet our kids with questions like, *Did you brush your teeth? Make your bed? Get all your homework done?* Without realizing it, you may be asking questions that convey *conditional* approval or love. Your child has many things that are good about them. They don't have to do anything to have value. They don't need to be thinner to be worthy. They don't need to be smarter to be precious. They don't have to be taller or muscular to be valuable. They don't have to be popular to be important. They are worthy *as is*. Because they *exist*, they deserve love, food, and care.

> **#TruthBomb:**
> Directly and indirectly, children with larger or smaller bodies may get the message they aren't worthy. Over time, this can turn into self-loathing, the opposite of self-love.

Self-Esteem: I Achieve

As you've learned, self-esteem is built through skill development, validation, and nurturing. Where worthiness is a given, regardless of what your child has done or achieved, self-esteem is tied to your child's accomplishments and qualities. When your child feels valuable, self-esteem can follow. Higher self-esteem boosts performance, a sense of well-being, and personal growth, and provides a buffer against setbacks and failures. Children who feel capable and confident are happier. Low self-esteem, on the other hand, produces the opposite effect: disinterest in learning, negative feelings like anger and sadness, withdrawal and difficulty making friends, and the tendency to bend to peer pressure and use self-defeating coping mechanisms like too much screen time, overeating, and other avoidance tactics. Lower self-esteem may even lead to a dislike of self. Self-esteem may decline as kids age and when their body and self-image waver. Being bullied, too much academic or social stress, or negative feedback can erode it, too. Gender, school performance, socio-economic status, parent education, and employment are additional factors that may contribute to lower self-esteem.

Self-Care: I Nurture Myself

Self-care is how we care for ourselves, physically and emotionally. It's those things we do to keep ourselves well, like getting enough sleep, eating, moving, and taking breaks when we need them. It can include whom you choose to spend time with and what you view and consume on social media. Self-care has several benefits to those who practice it, such as reduced anxiety and depression, lowered stress, more energy, less burnout, and better relationships.

The act of self-care, whether it be getting to bed on time, having some alone time to read, or taking a relaxing bath, sends the message that you care about yourself and your well-being. Taking the time to celebrate accomplishments, surrounding yourself with encouraging friends, acknowledging your feelings and needs, and setting boundaries all point to caring for oneself, too, reinforcing worthiness and value.

Self-Care Ideas

Physical Self-Care	Emotional Self-Care	Mental Self-Care
Get to bed on time	Laugh	Journal thoughts and emotions
Move every day, outside as much as possible	Cry	Read
Take a bath	Give thanks	Meditate
Breathe deeply	Speak kindly to yourself	Take a social media break
Nap	Self-soothe	Follow a daily routine
Make delicious food	Hang out with positive people	Create goals and celebrate achieving them
Dance	Light a candle	Set clear boundaries and expectations
Get or give yourself a massage	Pause and notice your surroundings	Challenge yourself to learn something new
Create a physical space that is nurturing	Compliment others and reflect on compliments you receive	Talk with a friend

PARENT STRESS AND SELF-CARE

A 2021 study found that adults who perceived more stress participated in fewer self-care activities. Unfortunately, many parents busy themselves with caring for their families and neglect their own needs. Tired all the time? Constantly worried or annoyed? Poor sleep? No time to fix yourself something to eat? These are signs of neglecting yourself. If this is you, please know it will be difficult to model and teach your child self-care practices. Many adults don't know how to care for themselves because they were never taught to do it as children. Here's your chance to change that and start a self-care journey. You won't gain martyrdom by sacrificing your needs. Fill your cup first. Only then can you fill the cup of your child and others.

Self-Awareness: I Know Myself

Self-awareness is being able to see yourself—your thoughts and feelings—and how they connect to your behaviors. You can build self-awareness in your child by making connections between their feelings and their behaviors, like helping them understand that being ignored by their friend may be why they want to eat or go to their room and watch videos. Or being nagged to try new foods at their grandparents' house is why they lost their appetite. It's connecting the feeling of shame when picked last on the playground to aggressiveness toward a sibling after school. Help your child understand, connect, and process their feelings to build their self-awareness.

Additionally, being self-aware helps your child control their behaviors. Understanding tendencies, like negative emotions triggering a desire to eat or exercise, gives us a moment to reflect and decide on our behavior rather than engage mindlessly. This can result in better decision-making, particularly if your child tends to engage in less-than-healthy behaviors. Self-knowledge may boost self-acceptance, encourage personal growth, and encourage initiative. In a study of medical students, self-awareness led to more self-care, and in law students, understanding one's own capabilities boosted emotional intelligence, or the ability to recognize and regulate emotions in ourselves and others.

Today, we have to take an active part in teaching our kids how to love themselves. This can't be a hollow or forgotten lesson. Not in today's world. We have to model this for them, talk about how to do self-care, and connect the dots to better feelings, emotions, and behaviors. Before we dig in to how to do this, let's explore some of the barriers that stand in your way. I'll be focusing on three main areas: disrespect, disempowerment, and disembodiment.

Takeaways:

- Self-love is a key to better mental health, self-acceptance, self-esteem, self-awareness, and motivation.
- Self-love is built from self-value, self-esteem, self-care, and self-awareness.
- Many parents don't know how to self-love, making it harder to cultivate it in their children.

OBSTACLES AND OBJECTIONS
It's All About the "Dis"

Positive experiences, support, and love during childhood fertilize the seeds of self-love. But families can be messy, and although mostly well-intentioned, they may not rise to their potential or provide what a child needs. And then there's our society. Norms, ideals, and prejudices are the weeds threatening to choke out the roots of self-love. From body size and appearance norms to social platforms and policies, societal pressures may undermine and call into question the good work of parenting and the family system. The two most powerful influences on your child's ability to love themself are rooted in family and society. Let's dive deeper and investigate how they make their mark on your child.

Disrespect, Disempowerment, and Disembodiment

The definition of disrespect is *a lack of regard or respect for*. The "for" part can be directed toward anything—humans, animals, plants, the planet, or an idea. We see disrespect in the home, workplace, classroom, health-care system, and political arenas. Disrespect, in general, causes the recipient to feel shame, anger and confusion, self-doubt, and a host of other feelings. When a child is raised in a disrespectful home or encounters disrespect, they can feel unworthy and unloved. This can taint how they see themself, affecting their future relationships and undermining the development of self-love.

As I reviewed in Pillar One, disrespect in the home may be demonstrated by criticism and shaming a child about their body size or eating, belittling their ideas or accomplishments, and ignoring their needs. Disrespect targeting size is a form of oppression and prejudice. Some adults will size-discriminate under a shroud of showing concern and care. *I'm on her case because I worry about her health down the road. I foresee a future of teasing, and I don't want that for him. We have a history of heart attacks in our family, and I want to prevent that.* Of course, no parent wants their child to grow up with a likelihood of developing a chronic health condition or being teased, bullied, or discriminated against. But while a concern for "good health" is admirable and perhaps justified, when it comes to body size, it can be a smokescreen for bias and prejudice.

#TruthBomb: "Skinny is healthier" and "Fat is unhealthy" are biases, not evidence-based facts.

Of course, you want to help your child grow up healthy—physically *and* emotionally. That's why you're reading this book! And, yes, the parenting you do today sets your child up for behaviors tomorrow. But if all these good intentions for a future of health and well-being are bundled up in bias, bigotry, and oppression, they will only disrespect your child, undermine their value, and create obstacles to self-love and self-respect. Size discrimination can be subtle, and you may not recognize it in yourself, or in arenas like health care, but it often shows up like this:

- Commenting about a child's body and calling it a "joke."
- Talking about others' bodies (negatively or positively).

- Allowing family members to make fun of a child's or other people's bodies.
- Assuming body size is a choice, reflecting some higher or lower moral or personal value.
- Making assumptions about a person's character, ability, or value based on their size.
- Viewing leanness as a sign of success, self-control, happiness, or genetic superiority.
- Hiding or restricting foods that are fattening, high-calorie, or considered indulgent.
- Critiquing food choices and how much is eaten.
- Treating a child who is larger or smaller differently from others.

Check yourself. Be on the lookout for the moral high ground around thinness and appearance. The consequences of this affect us as parents as well as our kids, regardless of their size. Be self-compassionate and give compassion to your child and others. Think about how your own language and messages, especially around health and health-oriented behaviors, may affect your child. Do you have prerequisites about what it means to be "healthy" or "good enough?" You didn't create a world that emphasizes appearance, but make sure you're not perpetuating it.

> **#WiseAdvice:**
> Leanness and appearance are not prerequisites for respect.

Disrespect not only erodes self-esteem but can *disempower* an individual, or prevent them from having power, authority, or influence. Our culture attaches moral values and preferences to individuals who meet societal norms, what Jodi Pfarr, author of *The Urgency of Awareness*, calls a "normalized dominant identity." Our world is geared toward, and offers benefits to, those who have a normalized dominant identity, such as trim and fit, right-handed, educated, middle-to-upper class, and a slew of other identities. Having a normalized dominant identity allows access, voice, and a positive experience for the individual.

Children with larger and smaller bodies may be disempowered by a society that believes in an ideal body size. When a child's (or adult's) body size doesn't match this ideal, they may be considered "lesser"—less important, less valuable, and less influential. Their thoughts, ideas, and opinions matter less. Their experience in the world may be marginalized and different from those with normalized body types. Disempowerment can happen across the board—in classrooms, churches, health-care offices, and just about everywhere your child goes.

Disempowerment creates a barrier to well-being and health care. For example, weight-loss diets or exercise programs designed to "shrink" or help your child "grow better" may reflect societal norms ("bodies that are too big or too small are unacceptable and need to be fixed") rather than target a health condition. If your child is benched in sports or singled out to do different activities in gym class, underlying this may be the idea that "size dictates value." This bias disempowers you and your child while perpetuating the norms around appearance and size. How can you be empowered to raise your child, no matter their size, when you're faced with structures, systems, and ideologies that disempower you from the start? Short answer: you can't.

THE RISK OF DISEMBODIMENT

When any child is disrespected and disempowered due to their size, they're at risk for disembodiment—an intense disconnect from the mental, emotional, and physical aspects of their bodies. They aren't *present* in their body. When kids disconnect from their bodies, their ability to recognize and appreciate their body's needs is diminished. Furthermore, they're at risk for *believing* what society says—they are lazy, gluttonous, and irresponsible or weak, unhealthy, and a "problem." This can lead to self-loathing and an uptick in mental health concerns. In other words, size stigma gets "under the skin" and causes mental and physical consequences. Shockingly, simply *perceiving oneself as larger (or smaller) than acceptable by societal standards* can worsen health and well-being.

Shame and Its Triggers

When I was in first grade, my teacher, a nun, told the second-grade teacher (who was also a nun) in front of our class that I was "a talker," and it was doubtful I'd make it into second grade. Her public prediction was deeply embarrassing, and effective. I became afraid of speaking up in class . . . for years. I'd be the last to raise my hand. My report card would have comments like "I'd like to hear more from Jill in class." Not only did this early experience shade my confidence in communicating my own needs to others, it strangled my voice and my confidence in championing the ideas that mattered to me.

Guilt and shame are self-conscious emotions. They're experienced when a moral or social standard is violated or noticed by other people and may cause a child to negatively evaluate themself. When children make a mistake or don't measure up to norms or their own expectations, they may feel shame or guilt. These feelings are reinforced by disapproval from others and are felt as rejection. Guilt and shame aren't the same, however. Guilt comes from *doing* something wrong. *I feel guilty that I ignored my friend on purpose. I feel guilty that I was late for class. I feel guilty for sneaking cookies.* Regret, wishing things were different, and wanting to correct misdeeds generally follow guilt. Shame, on the other hand, is the feeling of *being* something wrong. *I'm smaller than everyone in my class. I'm too big. I'm not smart enough. I'm a talker. I'm bad because I like cookies.* Shame is characterized by feelings of worthlessness, powerlessness, and the desire to disappear, defend, or avoid.

Guilt and shame are also "social emotions." They guide us through our day-to-day lives and help us "get along" or "get ahead." They hold us back before we speak up or out of turn, do something socially unacceptable, or are something we feel is unacceptable. Self-conscious emotions differ from basic emotions in that they require self-awareness and the ability to differentiate self from others, which emerges in early toddlerhood. From age eight years on, most kids have felt guilt and shame and understand them.

Mild Shame versus Toxic Shame

A child naturally feels mild shame when they do something that falls outside of the norm, like loudly interrupting a conversation between adults. Parents may correct their child with love and support, and explain and redirect them to appropriate behavior. The child experiences mild shame but feels connected and learns. But when a parent consistently punishes or scolds a child for their missteps, the child may feel alone, defective, and not good enough. This is defined as "toxic shame." Toxic shame undermines confidence, discourages risk-taking, and has been associated with substance abuse. Furthermore, parents who experienced shame in childhood may pass it on to their children. For instance, if you grew up as a person who felt body shame, you may be triggered when you see your own child overeating in public or hear your doctor or family member say your child's too large (or too small). As a way to soothe your own feelings of shame, you may blame your child for their eating habits or size. It's your child's fault, not yours. Now, your child feels disconnected from you. They feel shame. And your shame has been passed along.

For some kids, the response to shame is to become perfect. To never make mistakes. To be a "good" girl or boy. To change the way they behave or look. This drive to be perfect may turn into anxiety and depression (because perfection is impossible to achieve). Toxic shame may also turn a child into an angry kid, resisting a parent's guidance and becoming defiant. The bottom line: toxic shame is inconsistent with self-love.

Negative Feedback Is a Powerful Shame Trigger

The feedback your child gets from others helps them develop their social emotions. Adults give both positive and negative feedback to children, which helps them understand the "rules of the road" and how to navigate that road so they can be successful. *Positive* feedback is tied to feelings of happiness and pride, both positive emotions, while *negative* feedback is associated with emotions like sadness, shame, or guilt. What is negative feedback? Criticism, comments, and face-making, for instance. These can be perceived as a judgment of one's person or being. Character evaluations like *You love food too much*, *You're picky*, and *You're addicted to your phone*; teasing with pet names that call out size or physical abilities; or bullying that discriminates based on size, race, or gender identity, potentially assassinate the worthiness of a child. Believe it or not, this can happen as young as the preschool years. When heard over and over, a child's worthiness and ability to self-love erode like a sand dune in a hurricane. Negative feedback of any kind may be traumatic for any child, especially if it's given in public. Imagine living in a world where negative feedback, including harassment, bullying, and teasing, is served alongside an undercurrent of social rejection.

Social rank also affects feelings of guilt and shame. If a child perceives they are unpopular, this may change their self-worth and how they interact in groups. Kids who perceive themselves as disliked may behave submissively—avoiding eye contact, fear grinning (an indicator of emotional stress), and showing a lack of confidence, which is often accompanied by shame and guilt. Girls seem to be more susceptible to shame and guilt than boys, and *negative feedback* is one of the strongest triggers of guilt and shame in children.

It doesn't mean you can never provide feedback to your child. But you need to make sure feedback is targeting behaviors, not *who* your child *is*. Even then, it can trigger negative emotions about the self. Apologizing and repairing isolated incidents of negative feedback go a long way because kids are resilient. But if a child is hearing negative feedback about who they are or their body size, and it's coming from their loved ones at home, too, it can be overwhelming and potentially lead to a lifetime of numbing out—overeating, too much screen time, and perfectionism.

I'm not going to Pollyanna self-love and make you think if you do steps one, two, and three, you can raise a child who has self-love and everything will be all right. No, you're up against a societal reality, deeply embedded and reinforced in every medium we engage with and absorb. Self-love is not something you can guarantee. But it's not something you should gamble on, either. You've got a mountain to climb. You must climb it because you are the most important individual in your child's life, and your home is the safest place they can be. So don your mountain boots, crampons, and helmet, and get ready for the climb.

······················ **Takeaways:** ·····················

- Disrespect may occur anywhere, causing negative self-evaluations and feelings of unworthiness and blocking the ability to self-love.

- Bias about body size interferes with respect and the unconditional love of a child. Worse still, it's steeped into our social structures, systems, and ideologies, potentially disempowering children with larger and smaller bodies.

- Shame is triggered by negative feedback and is a barrier to self-love.

HOW TO STRIVE AND THRIVE
Cultivate Self-Love at Every Size

It's not unusual to hear adults talk about self-care. They talk about "me time," or embark on a journey of self-acceptance. In a way, it's an awakening experience to realize that you are who you are. Acceptance leads to more happiness than continually rejecting yourself. This later recognition may be accompanied by regret: *I wish I would've appreciated my body more. I wish I would have been more adventurous. I wish I would have worn that bikini.* It's too bad that it takes many adults so long to get to this point. You have an opportunity to change this and jump-start intentional self-love for your child.

In this section, I will tie the Pillars of Wellness that you've already learned about to the development of self-love, explore some self-love practices you can implement with your child, and show you how to better advocate for your child (and others), making this world a better place for *every* child.

Integrate the Pillars of Wellness

If you've made it this far, you've learned how each Pillar of Wellness impacts your child's physical health and emotional well-being. You've learned how to tackle each Pillar based on where you're at right now. Perhaps it's clear how these Pillars build self-love. But for the purpose of completion, let's review each Pillar and connect it to your child's self-value, self-esteem, and self-love.

Family culture sets the tone for body acceptance, respect, and inclusivity. Role-modeling health behaviors, cultivating a safe, nurturing environment, and promoting family cohesion help your child grow up in a family that accepts one another, celebrates diversity in all bodies, and rejects negative influences. This forms a foundation of trust, worthiness, and self-esteem.

Sleep helps your child manage their energy, mood, and physical health. It repairs the body and mind, regulating body and brain functions and emotions. Sleep helps your child start the day feeling refreshed, ready, and regulated.

Movement helps your child be healthy and feel good. Movement encourages physicality and better mood, and raises self-esteem. It also helps your child *be* in their body—be embodied—and can increase your child's body appreciation and enjoyment.

Feeding helps your child build trust and connection with the family and develop a positive relationship with food and their body. It reinforces self-trust, autonomy, and agency over what goes into their body. Because feeding is something you do each day, it's a constant influencer on your child's ability to trust themself (and you!) with food.

Eating behaviors are developed during childhood and predict future eating habits. The goal is to establish self-regulation skills and use body feedback to govern food intake. When your child learns to self-regulate their eating, their self-trust and autonomy increase.

Food is essential to everyday life. Being flexible about food teaches your child they can enjoy all types of food without guilt or shame. Although the main job of food is to nourish your child, we must not forget that it does much more than that. It's a way to connect with others, regulate appetite and emotions, and build a healthy relationship with food and their body.

Screens and media increasingly sway your child's self-view by way of comparison. Although screens can be a positive mode of learning and even awareness of positive body messaging, screens are a looming threat to your child's sense of worthiness and self-love.

Active cultivation of self-love is a priority for every family raising a child, particularly for those raising children with larger or smaller bodies. Each one of these Pillars of Wellness plays a role in how your child feels about themselves and whether they actively care for their body and mind. Raising *any* child who is confident, self-compassionate, resilient, and self-advocating means implementing the Pillars advantageously.

Cultivating the habits in each Pillar *is* self-care. The goal here is to engage in health-promoting habits as an enjoyable path to self-care. Self-care rituals—such as enjoyable movement, a yoga class, meditation, breathing exercises, journaling, a relaxing bath in the middle of the day, an early bedtime, a screen break, an ice-cream cone for lunch, or time out to read a book—not only cement healthful behaviors, they're acts of self-love. It brings me joy when my twenty-four-year-old announces she's taking some "self-care time," which often means a nap or a bath in the middle of the day. She's learned that self-care is an important symbol of self-love.

Practical Self-Love Maneuvers

Self-love is cultivated over time, not overnight. Although you need to have your eye on the barriers to self-love, like body-shaming, disrespect, and other transgressions, you also need to encourage self-love practices your child can habituate to over time. You don't have to wait until your child is in their twenties to practice self-care.

Have Your Child Take "Me Time"

Put time on the calendar for self-care. Maybe it's once a month, once a week, or every day. The fact that it takes up space on the calendar means it's important. Create a list of "Me Time" activities such as getting a pedicure or painting nails, taking a bubble bath or a longer than usual shower, sleeping in, lighting a candle and reading, listening to music, meditating, cooking with an adult or independently, or taking an afternoon "lay me down." Don't forget to emphasize "Me Time" as a priority for self-care.

Journaling

Journaling encourages self-awareness and rewires the brain to think positively, especially when it centers on positive ideas and thoughts.

Encourage your child to keep a journal of their positive qualities and events each day. Maybe someone gave your child a compliment. Or they feel proud of how they treated someone. Journaling should emphasize *what is good about your child*. Home in on your child's strengths, talents, and how they treat others.

If your child is too young to journal on their own, consider an "I Love Me" journal jar. You can write down a positive attribute, action, or event on a slip of paper and place it in the jar for your child. Try to do this each day. If your child has a down day, pull out the jar and read the slips of paper. It will undoubtedly help them feel better.

Words of Affirmation

Positive comments about who your child is—their qualities and characteristics—affirm they are enough just as they are. Don't overinflate these or be hollow. Seek out what is true. Look for the positives in all areas—your child is kind, just, thoughtful, humorous, artistic, agile— and be specific. If these can flow from your mouth, they will come easily to your child when they are down or doubting their self-worth.

On the mirror

Write a message to your child on a sticky note and place it on the bathroom mirror. Examples: *You are prepared. I believe in you. I'm your biggest fan! You can be anything you want to be. I'm so proud of you. I love that you never give up.*

In the lunch box

Send a message to your child in their lunch box. A lunch box love note can be empowering, encouraging, and loving. Examples: *You are a good friend. You make the world better. I like how your mind works. You are learning something new each day. You are an amazing creature! Remember, I love you. There's only one of you and I'm so glad you're mine.*

At the meal table

Use the family meal table to converse about "One Good Thing" that happened that day. Go around the table and have everyone share a comment or experience from the day. Example: "Ted said I was his best friend today," said a six-year-old child. "Why do you think Ted said that?" asked his dad. "Because I always sit with him at lunch," said the child. Dad takes time to reflect on what it means to be loyal and a good friend, affirming his son has these qualities.

Advocacy and Activism: Justice for Bodies of Every Size

Acceptance of your child, no matter their size, is essential to raising a child who loves themselves. But this is only the beginning. You will need to take this further if you want to change the world in which your child is growing up. Being an advocate for your child and others, and raising awareness of size bias and discrimination, will go a long way to furthering body dignity for children of every size.

Show your child that you *actively* accept other bodies, just like you might advocate for racial or religious acceptance. Eradicate the idea that everyone can have the same body size. It's defeating, destructive, and an ideology. Here are some ways to be an advocate for all bodies.

Call out unfair or unequal treatment. When your child is picked (or not) for a role in a play, a position on the team, or another activity based on appearance, not ability, call it out for what it is: discrimination. Take the opportunity to kindly educate adults who perpetuate unequal treatment based on size or appearance. Encourage your child to also be an agent of change.

Encourage your child to set boundaries. Replying to Grandma with a polite "no" to extra helpings of food engages self-advocacy and autonomy. Empower your child to stand up for themselves with their peers and other discriminating adults. Teach them to reply with *"That's not cool,"* or *"That's mean,"* and immediately walk away when another person bullies or shames their body. Give your child permission to have the last word and disengage. Tell your child that when others bully or shame them (or someone else), it's more about the bully than it is about your child.

Fill your social media feed with #BoPo (body positivity) messaging and follow groups on social media that advocate for body diversity and people of all shapes, sizes, colors, genders, and abilities. You can find body positivity messaging on social media by searching the hashtags #BoPo, #bodyneutrality, #bodypositivity, #bodypositive, #bodyacceptance, #allbodiesaregoodbodies, and #selflove.

Speak to health and body function, not appearance or thinness. Use body-neutral language, like *Your healthy lungs help you breathe deeply and relax, Your legs take you where you need to go,* or *Your smile lights up a room!* Steer clear of expressions like *"lose weight," "trim down," "buff up,"* and *"get fit,"* which can stigmatize and make children feel bad or less than.

Expose your child to kids of all sizes, colors, genders, religious beliefs, and abilities. Promote engagement with positive people who care about them, have good character, and act like good friends in their lives.

Focus on the whole child. Your child is so much more than their body size. You can never say this enough!

While you may not have imagined you would be an activist for all bodies, this is your next move. It is what needs to happen for your (and every) child to grow up in a world that accepts them for who they are, not what they look like. Accepting your child is where you begin, but being an advocate and activist for size diversity is where societal change happens, promoting the next generation of kids who are healthy *and* feel good about who they are, no matter their size.

THE WHOLE-CHILD CHECKUP
Self-Love

Realistically, your child will grow up with moments of loving themselves and moments of serious self-doubt and dislike. These ups and downs will exist, as they have for generations before. And although you cannot guarantee self-love, you can do your part to nudge its development. Let's check in on how you're doing right now and outline your next steps. Are you a Learner, Striver, or Thriver?

The Learner: Where Do I Begin?

Let's be honest—your head may be spinning right now. Advocacy? Activism? Others of you may be saying, "Yes, bring it on!" Because you've been reading this book, you know the Pillars of Wellness help you raise not only a physically healthy child, but one who feels good about themself. Keep working your way through each Pillar so you can set up the best environment for your child as they grow. Remember, each Pillar informs and influences your child's developing sense of self and self-appreciation.

Keep shaping body-neutral language. Use words that describe bodies like *strong* or *flexible*, and comments about people such as *having a caring attitude*, *being a loyal friend*, or *being responsible*. Focus on character and body function, not on form or appearance.

I also recommend a deeper dive into how societal norms and ideology influence your child's feelings about themself and others. Remember, society works well for some of us, and not so well for others. If your child is an "other" because they're growing up in a larger or smaller body, or have different abilities or challenges, then learning more about injustice and inequality in our culture will strengthen advocacy for your child. I have a few resources in the Appendix.

The Striver: Let's Level Up

At this level, you're practicing all the Pillars every day and working to ingrain habits. If you encounter negative body talk—within your family or outside your home—your goal is to eradicate it. Your work here is to teach others what you've learned about body diversity and promoting dignity for all children. Develop quick one-liners you can use, like *All bodies are good bodies and we prefer to focus on our child's qualities and characteristics, not their appearance*. Or *Our child is [characteristic or quality]—we focus on the inside qualities in our family, not the outside ones*. Invite conversations about your values around body size and diversity. You'll show your child support and help others think differently and, hopefully, act differently.

Encourage your child to speak up for themself or others when faced with size discrimination, no matter their size. Role-play different scenarios, and act out what they could do and say to self-defend or stick up for a friend. Not only does this equip your child for tricky situations, it also boosts their confidence in handling them.

Self-Love: Learner, Striver, or Thriver

	Learner	Striver	Thriver
Pillars of Wellness	Parent is in the beginning stages of implementing all the Pillars. Baby steps are in progress! Returns to each Pillar chapter to outline goals and keep moving forward.	All Pillars are engaged. Making strides in each area and making the connection of self-care to self-love.	Family is doing well in each Pillar. Time for self-care is part of the weekly schedule.
Practical Self-Love Maneuvers	Self-care is a new concept. Parent is familiar with self-care but hasn't tried it for themselves. Hasn't encouraged this with the child yet.	Self-care time is on the schedule, albeit inconsistently. Encourages child to journal, move, and take "Me Time," though it's not part of the family routine. Positive feedback is given frequently.	Parent and child practice self-care and prioritize it. Self-love is a goal for each family member.
Advocacy and Activism	Parent isn't accustomed to being an activist, especially not for bodies. Tries suggestions for advocacy and activism on behalf of their child. Curious and interested in solving the dilemma of body stigma for all children. Understands societal norms around appearance are damaging.	Parent has advocated for their child, or other children. Parent feels empowered and wants to do more. These experiences have offered a pathway to healing old wounds for themselves. Child is encouraged to speak up, not shy away from bullies and unfair treatment.	Family is outspoken about body-shaming and discrimination. Empowers child to stand up for themselves and call out body bias. Advocates for equality, fair treatment, and dignity for all bodies. Child is confident, loves themselves, and regularly practices self-care.

The Thriver: Keep Up the Good Work

You are well on your way to actively cultivate self-love, while arming your child with the awareness, sensitivity, and kindness to treat others fairly and with compassion. If you have a child who has a larger or smaller body, you're raising them with dignity and respect. Undoubtedly, it's an uphill climb to raise a child who feels good about themself in today's world. But it's so worth the effort!

You're about to read the last chapter in this book, which contains the Size Wise Assessment, some parting wisdom, and some frequently asked questions (FAQs). Before you get there, I leave you with this:

Dear Size Wise Parent,

May you always love yourself, so you have abundant love for your child and others.

May you create a family culture of respect, acceptance, and dignity, so your child may respect themself and carry these qualities out into the world.

May you sleep deeply each night, so you greet your child (and the day) with patience, optimism, and fortitude.

May you delight in moving your body, so your child catches your enthusiasm.

May you feed and nourish yourself well, so you can nurture a positive relationship with food and eating within your child.

May you enjoy eating, so you can show your child one of life's greatest pleasures.

May you balance all foods, so you can nourish the mind, body, and soul of yourself and your child.

May you temper your engagement with screens, so your child learns to do so, too.

May you accept all bodies, no matter their size, so your child always feels accepted and accepts others.

May you embrace the goodness of all bodies and change the world for all children.

XO, Jill

It does not matter how slowly you go
so long as you do not stop.

—CONFUCIUS

....

Thriving at Every Size, Inside and Out

The Assessment and More

....

ongratulations! You've made it to the finish line. But it's only the beginning. You understand the importance of positive lifestyle behaviors, how they impact your child's health and well-being, and the guidance you need to get started. If you're doing the work, you may notice a happier, more relaxed, and more confident child; fewer struggles and questions; and a feeling that you have a promising path ahead, one that helps your child be both physically healthy and emotionally well. The future is bright.

Remember, much of your child's size is preprogrammed. Your efforts to establish good habits and support your child are important. You're cultivating a *lifestyle*, and it's a long game. Keep your eye on the prize: creating a connection and relationship with your child, and cultivating the habits that will serve them throughout their life.

You may also have a little voice in your head asking, *Will implementing these behaviors change my child's size?* It's normal to have this question.

Sizeism and its ideals are deeply embedded and hard to break from. Maybe there will be a noticeable change, or maybe not. This book was never intended to be a weight-loss or weight-gain plan. But through adopting positive lifestyle behaviors, you may see changes. More important, positive habits help your child grow up in the body they were designed to have, feel good about it, and improve their quality of life, now and later. If your child feels good, they'll be more likely to care for their body. If their body is functioning well, it's more likely they'll feel good. I urge you to think about your child from the Whole-Child Healthy perspective, always considering your child's physical health and emotional well-being. When there is too much focus on physical health, you run the risk of sacrificing emotional well-being. And the opposite is true—when emotional well-being becomes too centralized, you can lose sight of physical health. You need both to raise a healthy, happy child.

In this final chapter, you will be directed to the comprehensive Size Wise Assessment on page 246, summarizing all of the Pillars of Wellness so you have an overview at your fingertips. Knowing how you're doing at any point in time will help you stay on track. The Size Wise Assessment also provides a basis for talking about your child's health and well-being with your health-care provider. You'll also learn a simple method for addressing any habit you want to cultivate and find a question-and-answer section. Before we get there, though, I want to leave you with a few thoughts.

Influence what you can. Some things are predetermined, like your child's genetic tendency to be larger or smaller, carry more body fat, or have strong temperamental or appetitive traits. These aren't in your control. They're hard-wired. Consider these traits as you raise your child, and implement strategies that support their unique qualities and characteristics. For instance, if your child tends to be resistant, you'll want to collaborate with them and get their buy-in. If your child is food responsive, curate a food environment that isn't too tempting and hard for them to navigate. And if they carry more body fat naturally, pay more attention to buoying their worthiness, esteem, and emotional well-being.

There are many things over which you have influence, such as your family and food culture, your home environment, and your words, actions, and attitudes. This book has offered you ways to optimize key health and lifestyle behaviors and the other influences that shape your child's emotional well-being. Spend your time and effort on these rather than on the things you cannot control.

Accept and cherish the child you have. You may have a child who is naturally smaller, and always will be. Or larger-framed with a tendency to carry more body fat. Your child can't help the fact they inherited Grandpa's slight build or Aunt Sally's tummy, hips, and legs, any more than any other inherited quality, tendency, or condition, like curly hair or the predisposition to heart disease. The world today casts bias and stigma on those who don't fit into the constricted definition of appearance and health. No matter your child's size, don't align with these harmful societal ideologies. Remember, if you're not accepting your child, you're rejecting them.

All bodies need good habits. The 8 Pillars of Wellness aren't just for kids with larger or smaller bodies; they're for *all* kids. Don't make the mistake of believing your child doesn't need to develop good habits. They do. *Every* child does.

Parent for the long haul. Model the path to a healthful way of life. That's your parenting job and the heart of this book. Yes, you're on the hook through adolescence, but beyond that, it's up to your child to embrace and adopt these lifestyle behaviors. Although your child's engagement in healthful habits may vacillate over the years, you've carved the habit path. It's familiar, and there for the taking at any time. And that's a success.

Habits can change. The habits your child develops can be long-lasting. That's a double-edged sword—good or bad habits may take root. If you find yourself facing unhelpful habits, there's good news. Children are learners who are pliable and resilient, especially when they have loving parents guiding them.

Advocate for all children. Bias and discrimination may be more damaging than we know at this point in time. As mental health concerns are increasing, parents and adults need to step up and advocate for all children, challenging the societal norms around size and health. Can children be larger or smaller and healthy? Yes. Can they be emotionally secure and smaller or larger? Yes. But only if the world around them shifts away from negative assumptions, stigma, exclusion, and unfair treatment based on size.

Your child, your choice. You have the knowledge and skills to make the best choices for your child and family, based on your circumstances. If you need more information to make a sound decision, seek out health-care providers such as doctors, dietitians, and mental health counselors in your community who align with your family values and goals. You deserve to feel comfortable, confident, and empowered on your path. Tailor each Pillar to the needs of your child, your family, and your situation. There's no right or wrong path. There's just *your path*.

Are You Size Wise?

Together, the Whole-Child Healthy model and the 8 Pillars of Wellness have described what it takes to raise children of *every* size in today's world with sensitivity and practicality. The goal is for your child to grow up physically healthy and emotionally well, participating in enjoyable, healthful behaviors, and regulating them as they mature.

As a Size Wise parent or caregiver, you also have a basis for communicating with your health-care provider. For one, you can specify how you want your health-care provider to address any concerns they have about your child. I hope you will feel empowered to request private conversations about size or health concerns, at a minimum. These can be done on the phone or over email. No child should be present for these conversations. Additionally, you may make a note in your child's medical record asking health-care providers to not mention weight in front of your child, not weigh your child at every visit, and avoid "diet" talk or any other potentially stigmatizing topics in the presence of your child.

When speaking with your pediatrician, you might also share your knowledge and the work you're doing at home by saying, *"We're doing great with sleep hygiene and screen time, and working on food balance, movement, and our family culture."* Not only does this highlight the importance of behaviors (versus your child's size), but it also shows off your knowledge about the many influences on your child's health and emotional well-being. You might also say something like, *"We're actively working on self-care and body appreciation so our child knows they are loved as they are, no matter what."* Can you imagine the conversation that might ensue? I imagine a remarkable partnership with your health-care provider!

How to Build a Good Habit, Simplified

What if there's a habit you want to cultivate, but it's not covered in this book? When I wrote the *How-to* section of each Pillar chapter, I used a simple three-step method to attack building habits intentionally. You can adopt this approach for any habit you want to build.

Step 1: Identify the Case for Building a Habit

First, ask yourself, *Why do I want to create this habit?* For each Pillar, I looked at the research and summarized the case for building the lifestyle behavior. Although you don't need to do research, you do need to tap into the desire around building a habit. Why is it important to you, or to your child? What is the payoff?

Let's take school lunches as an example. Perhaps you want your child to have a homemade lunch a few days of the week. You'd like to get into the habit of assembling lunch the night before with your child—not right before they head out the door in the morning. Alternatively, if your child buys school lunch most days of the week, you may want to establish a habit of reviewing the school lunch menu with your child so they get a balanced, energizing meal in the middle of the day. You feel better knowing they're eating foods at lunchtime that are nutritious and fuel them for the day. That's your *why*.

Step 2: Acknowledge the Barriers

Obstacles and objections are the biggest barriers to building habits. In order for a habit to take hold, you must overcome the barriers and create an environment that makes repeatable behaviors *easy*. The second step is to identify the obstacles standing in your way.

Let's revisit our example. Some of the barriers to prepacking or preselecting lunch with your child might be: a later dinner due to family or work schedules; homework demands; a lack of lunch items available; you or your child being too tired or exhausted to connect around this topic; or evening commitments that remove you or your child from the home. These are your *obstacles*. By identifying these barriers, you can come up with a plan that skirts them, making the behavior easier to achieve and repeat.

Step 3: Identify a Simple Plan

Now that you know why you want to establish a habit and the barriers that potentially get in the way, break down the habit into simple, bite-size steps—a simple plan that directly addresses the barriers you've identified above. In our example, you may realize that assembling lunch or talking about tomorrow's school offerings after dinner won't work. Too many obstacles arise in the evening. Assembling tomorrow's lunch after school, while your child is eating their snack, or during dinner preparation would be better. Or preselecting school lunch over the weekend could work. Together with your child you decide when you'll pack or preselect lunch. For packing lunches, you talk about lunch items for the week, decide together and include them on your shopping list, and shop for them so they're available when it comes time to pack lunch. For lunch from school, you print out the school lunch menu and talk about the items your child will select during the week, circle them, and post the menu somewhere obvious as a reminder to both of you.

Once you've formulated a habit-building plan, get started with the behavior. When your child comes home from school and settles in with their snack, you may say, "Hey, what shall we pack for lunch tomorrow?" You both decide what lunch will be, pull out the items, assemble them together, put them in the lunch box, and store it for the next day. Voila! You've packed lunch with your child the day before. Or, on Sunday, you sit down for ten minutes with your child and select the week's lunch menu together. To build any habit, you'll want to repeat your simple plan often and soon a habit will form. You can apply this method to any habit you want to establish. The key is to make sure the habit is worth building, address the barriers, and repeat the behavior.

Frequently Asked Questions (FAQs)

I suspect you may have some questions about size extremes. Here, I point you to more help and some practical advice. No matter your child's size and situation, implementing *all* of the Pillars of Wellness that you've learned here will be expected and advised. There is no treatment or approach that leaves the Pillars of Wellness out of the process, especially if you want to keep a balanced focus on both health and well-being. My other books and my website, The Nourished Child, offer you more resources and direction should you have other questions about nutrition and feeding your child beyond the scope of *Kids Thrive at Every Size*. Additionally, I've selected a few more resources (located on page 242) should you want to keep learning.

How do I find a health-care provider who will be sensitive to my child's emotional well-being?

Size stigma, unfortunately, exists in health care. Two-thirds of adults who are larger in size and who report a past history of size stigma say it came from their doctors. It's not just doctors, though. It can be nurses, therapists, administrators, and, yes, dietitians. As a result, many individuals who may need more help avoid seeking it. Judgment, a lack of listening and respect, or the feeling they need to lose weight before seeing the doctor keep them from getting medical treatment.

The *weight-inclusive approach* mitigates the shame and stigma many people with larger bodies experience from the health-care system. It focuses on health and well-being as being multifaceted, not as outcomes of size, and prioritizes access to care and reducing size stigma. It aligns with what you've learned throughout this book— that health and well-being can be achieved no matter one's size and when nonstigmatizing health care is provided. In a weight-inclusive approach, changing size is not a focal point. Rather, behaviors such as eating, moving, and sleeping are centralized and modified so they are enjoyable and regular. Weight loss is not a priority, and blame for a lack of success in this area is not put upon the individual but on the problematic process of losing weight.

When seeking a weight-inclusive health-care professional, look for the following:

- A belief that bodies come in all shapes and sizes.
- An understanding of health as a multidimensional state.
- A focus on healthful behaviors rather than weight loss.
- A priority on process rather than an end result (achieving a certain BMI or size).
- Individualized advice tailored to your lived environment and your circumstances.
- Acknowledgment of access, autonomy, and social justice as influences on health and well-being.

Another way to identify a weight-inclusive health-care professional is to evaluate the environment and vibe of their office. Is there furniture for bodies of all sizes? Are children weighed and measured in private? Are the health concerns you're there for prioritized, or is there more attention placed on your child's size? If it's the latter, this is a sign that size is a primary focus: the opposite of a weight-inclusive professional experience. Remember, you get to choose how you want your child's health and size handled at a health-care professional's office. You can ask questions, offer resources (like this book!), and help change the structures and systems that may oppress children with larger or smaller bodies just by advocating for your own child.

My child is larger and getting bigger. What can I do?

"We have a nine-year-old who is above the 97 percentile on all his body measurements, and I have no idea how to get this situation under control," said Anita, a physician. "We've gone to the pediatrician, a specialty weight clinic, and a therapist and nothing is changing (in fact, it may be getting worse). I know the data and recommendations. Even I can't seem to live by them." If your child is growing faster than expected, you may wonder if you should be doing something different. As you've learned, size is a product of genetics and environment. You can't change the gene pool, but you can fine-tune the environmental influences over which you have control.

The first thing I, and any health-care provider, will advise you to do is implement *everything* you've learned here. Yes, every Pillar of Wellness. Even if you think you have, it's a good idea to check the Size Wise Assessment on page 246 and see how you're doing. There's a lot to do! *Kids Thrive at Every Size* is one of the first (maybe only) books to help you set up healthy lifestyle behaviors early on, but it's also a resource for you along the way should you need to revise or reset habits.

> **#TruthBomb:**
> Health conditions, like high blood pressure or high cholesterol, also occur in bodies that are smaller and mid-sized. The presence of health conditions (versus the size of your child) is most concerning for their overall health.

If your child is accumulating health conditions that compromise their physical functioning, such as prediabetes or mobility challenges, your health-care provider will likely advise a more aggressive intervention. This will be based on the severity of health conditions, and whether lifestyle interventions have been working or not. Called intensive health behavior and lifestyle treatment (IHBLT), this intervention is often the next step when your child's physical health is compromised.

IHBLT centers on improving lifestyle behaviors in children as young as two years, with the goal of reducing or arresting body fat gain, as well as improving any coexisting health conditions. "Intense" means you'll be meeting with a health-care provider who is actively helping you achieve positive lifestyle behaviors and monitoring your child's progress. In other words, you won't be doing this on your own. IHBLT is most successful when the whole family is involved, it's face-to-face, and at least twenty-six hours of education is provided over the course of three months to a year. This type of support may be found in medical centers, coordinated through a pediatrician's office, or included in a community program. One of the primary obstacles to

IHBLT is accessibility. Finding this kind of intensified help is not easy and can be expensive, not to mention time-consuming.

If your child is growing larger, your health-care provider may worry about their physical health. Medical treatment focuses on treating health conditions and improving lifestyle behaviors, but it is often paired with weight-loss efforts. As you've learned, changing a child's size has its own set of risks: weight cycling, weight regain, a higher risk of disordered eating and eating disorders, and a negative effect on their emotional well-being. Positive lifestyle behaviors are good for *everyone*, and working on them to improve physical functioning makes sense. However, they may or may not be enough to reverse your child's health conditions if those conditions are significant.

> **#TruthBomb:**
> Children with special health-care needs, such as autism spectrum disorder (ASD), attention-deficit/hyperactivity disorder (ADHD), developmental or physical disabilities, appetite traits that promote eating, or use of medications that promote weight gain, are at higher risk for health concerns compared to their peers. If you have a child with special health-care needs, you may need more support as you raise them.

If you find your child is not improving with IHBLT, more aggressive approaches may be offered. The path you choose for your child is *your decision*. Work closely with a trusted doctor and health-care team who are equally sensitive to your child's emotional well-being. Do your homework and seek supportive professionals who keep your child's emotional well-being on par with their physical health. Some medical professionals may not be trained in a weight-inclusive approach; however, they may work with a team of other health-care professionals who are, like a registered dietitian, psychologist, or other mental health provider. Be particularly wary of size-focused interventions, especially if your child is physically healthy, naturally larger, and growing well. Remember, body function over form matters most.

My child is smaller and isn't growing well (or is getting smaller). What can I do?

When children don't grow well or don't eat enough, it may make even the most relaxed parent concerned. If this is happening in a child who is smaller, the worry magnifies. Although there can be a number of reasons for why a child may not grow, or becomes smaller—such as a chronic health condition like gastrointestinal malabsorption or multiple food allergies—the most common reason that the child is not eating enough. Why do children not eat enough? Most often it's due to picky eating or disordered eating (which may or may not evolve into a full-spectrum eating disorder).

Before I dive into both of these, I'm going to reinforce the Pillars of Wellness as the best foundation for helping your child. Yes, smaller kids who aren't growing well need good sleep, food, supportive interactions, movement, and more—all the Pillars you've already learned. It's easy to get focused on your child's size, or their eating, but I caution you. Overemphasizing size or eating runs the risk of problematizing your *child*, which may impact their mental health, leading to poor self-esteem and feelings of unworthiness.

Picky eating is a common rite of passage in toddlerhood. Most picky eaters grow well, and there's no need to make an issue of their eating behaviors or body size. But if your child's growth, health, body function, or emotional well-being are suffering, they may have an extreme form of picky eating, a condition called Avoidant/Restrictive Food Intake Disorder (ARFID), and need more support.

Changes in what, when, and how much your child eats, restrictive eating (e.g., no sugar, no gluten, no carbs, no dairy), or weight fluctuations are unfortunately more common than ever in preteens. These are dysfunctional eating behaviors and may lead to an eating disorder. Ironically, disordered eating happens in children of *every* size, even kids with larger bodies. If you see these signs, no matter your child's size, you'll want to better understand what's going on, so you can seek out the right support.

Extreme Picky Eating and ARFID

In the child who hasn't rolled through the toddler picky-eating phase smoothly, there may be underlying reasons, including mechanical concerns (e.g., a swallowing problem due to enlarged tonsils or adenoids); medical conditions (e.g., eosinophilic esophagitis); sensory sensitivities (off-putting characteristics of food like smell or texture); parental feeding dynamics (e.g., pressure to eat); behavioral aspects

#TruthBomb: Picky eating is highly heritable. It exists on a spectrum with developmental picky eating at one end and Avoidant Restrictive Food Intake Disorder (ARFID) at the other, and varying degrees and reasons for pickiness in the middle.

(e.g., anxiety); or a combination of these. As a result, some children may have ongoing struggles with food selectivity, affecting their social-emotional development, growth, and nutritional status. Whether your child needs more support will depend on the reasons for their pickiness and how it's affecting their health and quality of life.

When any child is shying away from the very sustenance that keeps them healthy and well, the inclination is to do everything you can to get your child to eat, but this, as you've learned, can backfire, making things much worse. This is the reason why most advice for developmentally expected picky eating will suggest a hands-off approach, encouraging you to let your child figure out their eating. But in children who are getting smaller, who may have nutritional deficiencies, or who experience a negative emotional impact on their quality of life, sensitive support can help.

First, why is your child fussy about food? Are they sensitive to certain characteristics of food? Is there an obstruction making swallowing uncomfortable? Is there too much pressure to eat or catering to food preferences? Figuring out the underlying causes of picky eating, especially the medical, mechanical, sensory, and feeding aspects, will direct the treatment path and identify the team of professionals, such as a pediatric dietitian, speech-language pathologist, occupational therapist, mental health counselor, or doctor. Depending on the underlying cause or causes—it can be multifactorial—the goal is to ease and alleviate these, as briefly outlined below.

#TruthBomb: In children with ARFID, nearly half say they are afraid of choking or vomiting, and a fifth report they avoid food due to sensory issues.

Medical Conditions: The goal is to treat any complicating medical problem, such as food allergies, eosinophilic esophagitis (a condition in which white blood cells build up in the esophagus, causing irritation, esophageal narrowing, and a sense of choking or food getting stuck), or gastrointestinal conditions.

Mechanical Problems: Chewing and swallowing can be difficult for some children, causing them to eat less. Treatment approaches are aimed at overcoming mechanical barriers to eating, like strengthening oral-motor skills to improve eating efficiency.

Sensory Sensitivities: Food characteristics like texture, odor, or flavor can dissuade a child from tasting and eating food. The goal here is to desensitize the child to the off-putting characteristics through gentle, repeated exposure to them.

Feeding Dynamics: Pressuring your child to eat or taste foods, using sweets to incentivize eating, and catering meals and snacks to a child's food preferences strengthen the push-pull feeding interaction between parent and child, often resulting in a child eating less. Supporting positive feeding interactions is the goal.

Behavioral Interventions: Some children are naturally more anxious and this shows up with eating. Some may demonstrate emotional reactions to disliked or unfamiliar foods, and other children may have other behaviors, like obsessive-compulsive disorder (OCD), in regard to eating. The goal is to ease these behaviors with therapeutic interventions from a qualified mental health counselor.

When a child needs more support for picky eating, the goal is to expand the diversity of the diet, improve growth and nutritional status, and build more confidence, adventure, and joy with eating. If your child is getting smaller and you suspect they need more help, talk with your health-care provider and jointly come up with a plan that considers both the health and well-being of your child.

Disordered Eating and Eating Disorders

It's estimated that about 13 percent of preteens and teens will develop an eating disorder, including anorexia, bulimia, or binge eating, by the time they turn twenty. Eating disorders have a genetic basis, too, and are the third most common chronic condition affecting teens. They can occur in children of *every* size, ethnicity, and gender.

Eating disorders start with disordered eating, with a fixation on appearance, body dissatisfaction, and a poor body image. "We think about eating disorders as a relatively rare occurrence," says Dr. Kendrin Sonneville. "But disordered eating is rampant." Ironically, parents often miss the signs of disordered eating, mistaking them for a positive change in eating behavior ("healthier eating"), dismissing them ("going through a picky eating stage"), or not recognizing them as problematic or probable (like not recognizing when boys have symptoms of disordered eating).

Here are some warning signs of disordered eating:

- Eating in secret
- Skipping meals or heading to the bathroom after eating
- Hoarding food
- Increased interest in calories, carbs, or other nutrients; or exercise
- Avoiding certain foods or food groups (carbs, processed foods)
- Weight fluctuations
- Expressed guilt or anxiety about eating or exercise

The best antidote to an eating disorder is to identify and treat disordered eating early. Treatment for disordered eating involves changing the mindset and thinking about food and the body. Often this may happen with a therapist who offers cognitive behavioral therapy (CBT), which helps individuals understand how their thinking influences their behavior. Work is done to change thoughts and behaviors.

#TruthBomb: Even moderate dieting makes a preteen or teen *five times* more likely to develop an eating disorder, and extreme food restriction makes them *eighteen times* more likely compared to teens who don't diet.

Acceptance and commitment therapy (ACT) is a form of CBT that helps people accept their thoughts and behaviors and get them to a more flexible place of thinking. Dialectical behavior therapy (DBT), also a type of CBT, encourages building new skills, regulating emotions, and tolerating stress using mindfulness and acceptance. Each of these approaches has similar goals: to address the thoughts behind disordered eating behaviors and ultimately change behaviors that may

EATING DISORDERS, BRIEFLY DEFINED

Anorexia nervosa (AN): Fear of becoming bigger; low body weight; avoiding or restricting food; body dysmorphia (experiences body differently from reality).

Bulimia nervosa (BN): Repeated episodes of eating a large amount of food generally within two hours; a sense of loss of control with eating; purging (vomiting, excessive exercise).

Binge-eating disorder (BED): Repeated episodes of eating without purging; loss of control; distress about eating.

ARFID: Extreme limits on types and amounts of food eaten; no fear of becoming bigger or distress about body size or shape.

Other specified feeding or eating disorder (OSFED): Significant eating difficulties that do not meet the criteria for AN, BN, BED, or ARFID.

push children along the spectrum of eating disorders. "I think of eating disorders existing on a spectrum," says Sonneville. "How much are you moving toward these clinically diagnosable eating disorders?"

If your child develops a full-spectrum eating disorder, treatment depends on the health and well-being of your child. When children are physically and psychiatrically stable, less intensive interventions, like outpatient therapy or partial hospitalization, are advised. If your child is medically compromised or their mental health is unstable, treatment may involve a residential or inpatient hospital stay. Family-based treatment is a home-based approach that's effective in children and teens with anorexia and bulimia, and potentially in children with ARFID. The focus is on refueling the body with food and restoring the child to a physically healthy state. Family members are considered an essential part of treatment, and play a big role in interrupting disordered eating and re-establishing nutritious and nurturing eating behaviors.

The good news is, everything you've learned in this book helps to prevent disordered eating and eating disorders. But despite having all the Pillars of Wellness in place and doing everything "right," some kids will develop one. That's because eating disorders are complex and multifactorial. Be extra vigilant if your child has a family history of eating disorders, or experiences high expectations to look a certain way, as they are at the highest risk. Don't get too hung up on why an eating disorder happened; rather, focus on getting the help your child needs as soon as possible, so they can recover as quickly as possible.

Remember, being smaller isn't necessarily a problem. But if your smaller child is getting smaller, or their eating behaviors set off alarm bells in your head, reach out to your health-care provider and have a conversation. Getting sensitive, supportive help can ward off further physical and emotional complications down the road.

It's a Wrap!

Remember Ann and Peter from the Introduction? I recently caught up with Ann. "Peter, now a sophomore in high school, is in a very good place," she said. "You were so helpful to us during those critical years." What Ann had was a solid road map—the Pillars of Wellness and the Whole-Child Healthy model—which helped her navigate and cultivate positive lifestyle behaviors and attitudes over the years. As a result, Peter is a confident teen who's healthy and happy. Of course, every child, family, and chosen path will be different, but many families will see positive outcomes when they focus on lifestyle behaviors that center on physical health *and* emotional well-being.

As we end our journey together, I hope you've learned there's more to raising healthy, happy kids than good food and exercise. With knowledge, empowerment, and a reasonable road map, you can begin your journey, or reboot it, and continue the long game of practicing and improving on the habits your child needs for a lifetime of health and well-being. Thank you for allowing me to join you on this part of your parenting journey. I wish you continued positive progress with your child. And now you can proudly state you are Size Wise!

APPENDIX

The Food Groups and Their Nutrients

Food Group	Nutrients
Protein	Iron, zinc, B vitamins (niacin, thiamin, riboflavin, B_6, and B_{12}), vitamin E, and magnesium. Omega–3 fats are found in fish and other seafood, and in nuts and seeds.
Grains	Grains, especially whole grain types, serve up fiber; B vitamins (thiamin, riboflavin, niacin, and folate), iron, magnesium, and selenium.
Dairy	Calcium, vitamin D, vitamin A, potassium, phosphorus, and protein.
Fruits	Vitamin C, fiber, potassium, and folate.
Vegetables	Vitamin A, vitamin C, fiber, potassium, and folate.
Fats and Oils	Vitamin E, omega–3 DHA, and omega–3 EPA. Solid fats include saturated and trans fats. Oils are a source of monounsaturated and polyunsaturated fat. Trans fats may be found in mayonnaise and salad dressing.

Examples	Comments
All meats such as poultry, beef, and pork; eggs; seafood; beans and peas; nuts and nut butter; and soy products.	Protein is also found in the dairy food group, and in small amounts in grains and some vegetables.
Any food made with wheat, rice, oats, barley, or other cereal grains, such as bread, crackers, cereal, pasta, rice, grits, and tortillas.	Two types of grains: whole grains and refined grains. A whole grain has its grain kernel intact, which means it carries fiber, like whole wheat bread. Refined grains like white bread are milled, meaning the bran and germ have been removed.
Milk, yogurt, cheese, and calcium-fortified soymilk.	Other dairy products like cream cheese or butter are not part of the dairy group. They fall into the fats and oils group. Plant-based milks, like almond milk, do not fall into this category because they lack adequate protein.
Apples and oranges, frozen berries, canned peaches, raisins, and 100% orange juice.	All fruits, including fresh, frozen, canned, dried, and 100% juice.
Red and orange vegetables: tomatoes, carrots, and sweet potatoes. *Dark-green vegetables*: romaine lettuce, spinach, and broccoli. *Starchy vegetables*: corn and potatoes. *Beans and peas* (also part of the protein group): pinto beans, black beans, black-eyed peas, kidney beans, and green peas. *Other vegetables*: onions, mushrooms, iceberg lettuce, green beans, and cauliflower.	All vegetables, whether fresh, canned, dried, frozen, or 100% juice; there are 5 subcategories: red and orange vegetables, dark-green vegetables, starchy vegetables, beans and peas, and other vegetables.
Solid fats: Butter, shortening, coconut oil, chicken fat, and lard. *Oils*: olive oil, canola oil, sunflower oil, vegetable oil, and corn oil. *Foods with oils*: nuts, olives, avocados, and some fish.	Some foods, like granola bars (which have fat as an added ingredient) or nuts (which are inherently fatty), already have fat included. Plant-based oils are heart healthy; solid fats contribute saturated fat and trans-saturated fats, both of which contribute to heart disease.

Daily Amounts for Food Groups and Starter Portions, Based on Age

Food Group	Daily Amounts and Starter Portions		
	3–4 years	**5–8 years**	**9–13 years**
Protein			
1 ounce = 1 egg; 1 ounce meat, fish, poultry	2–5 ounces per day	3–5½ ounces per day	4–6 ounces per day (girls); 5–6½ ounces per day (boys)
Beef, poultry, fish	1–2 ounces	2 ounces	3 ounces
Beans (cooked)	1–2 tablespoons	¼ cup	¼ cup
nuts, seeds	¼ ounce	½ ounce	½ ounce
nut butter	1–2 teaspoons	1 tablespoon	1 tablespoon
Egg	½–1	1	1
Grains			
1 ounce = ½ cup cooked grain; 1 slice bread; 5 whole wheat crackers; 1 cup cold cereal; 3 cups popcorn	3–5 ounces per day	4–6 ounces per day	5–7 ounces per day (girls); 5–9 ounces per day (boys)
Bread, bagel	¼–½ slice	1 slice, ½ bagel	1 slice, ½ bagel
Cold cereal	½ cup	1 cup	1 cup
Cooked cereal, pasta, rice	¼–½ cup	½ cup	½ cup
Crackers	2–3	5–6	5–7
Dairy			
1 cup milk, yogurt = 1½ ounces of cheese = ⅓ cup shredded cheese = 2 cups cottage cheese	2–2½ cups per day	2½ cups per day	3 cups per day

Food Group	Daily Amounts and Starter Portions		
	3–4 years	5–8 years	9–13 years
Dairy *(continued)*			
Milk, yogurt	½–¾ cup	¾–1 cup	1 cup
Cheese	½ ounce	¾–1 ounce	1½ ounce
Fruits			
	1–1½ cups per day	1–2 cups per day	1½–2 cups per day
Whole, fresh	1 cup	1 cup	1 cup
Cooked, canned	⅓ cup	½ cup	1 cup
Dried	¼ cup	½ cup	½ cup
100% fruit juice	½ cup	½ cup	1 cup
Vegetables			
	1–2 cups per day	1½–2½ cups per day	1½–3 cups per day (girls); 2–3½ cups per day (boys)
Whole, fresh	½ small	½–1 cup	1 cup
Raw, leafy greens	¼–½ cup	1 cup	1–2 cups
Cooked, canned	2–3 tablespoons	¼–1 cup	1 cup
100% vegetable juice	¼–⅓ cup	½ cup	½ cup
Fats and Oils			
Butter, margarine	1 teaspoon	1 teaspoon	1 teaspoon
Oil	1 teaspoon	1 teaspoon	1 teaspoon
Salad dressing, mayonnaise	1–2 teaspoons	1 tablespoon	1–2 tablespoons

Adapted from "Choose My Plate," U.S. Department of Agriculture, choosemyplate.gov

Additional Resources

THE BUILDING BLOCKS OF HEALTH

Clear, James. *Atomic Habits: Tiny Changes, Remarkable Results: An Easy & Proven Way to Build Good Habits & Break Bad Ones.* New York: Avery, 2018.

Segar, Michelle. *The Joy Choice: How to Finally Achieve Lasting Changes in Eating and Exercise.* New York: Hachette Go, 2022.

PILLAR ONE: Family Culture

Child Mind Institute: childmind.org/education

The Full Bloom Project: fullbloomproject.com

van der Kolk, Bessel. *The Body Keeps the Score: Brain, Mind and Body in the Healing of Trauma.* New York: Penguin Books, 2015.

Clarke-Fields, Hunter. *Raising Good Humans: A Mindful Guide to Breaking the Cycle of Reactive Parenting and Raising Kind, Confident Kids.* Oakland: New Harbinger, 2019.

Kennedy, Becky. *Good Inside: A Guide to Becoming the Parent You Want to Be.* New York: Harper Wave, 2022.

PILLAR TWO: Sleep

Sleep Education: sleepeducation.org

The Sleep Foundation: sleepfoundation.org/

Walker, Matthew. *Why We Sleep: Unlocking the Power of Sleep and Dreams.* New York: Scribner, 2017.

PILLAR THREE: Movement

Fit Kids: fitkids.org

Action for Healthy Kids: actionforhealthykids.org

PILLAR FOUR: Feeding

The Nourished Child: thenourishedchild.com

Ellyn Satter Institute: ellynsatterinstitute.org

Castle, Jill, and Maryann Jacobsen. *Fearless Feeding: How to Raise Healthy Eaters from High Chair to High School*, 2nd ed. Fearless Feeding Press, 2019.

Satter, Ellyn. *Child of Mine: Feeding with Love and Good Sense*. Boulder: Bull Publishing, 2000.

PILLAR FIVE: Eating

Tribole, Evelyn, and Resch, Elyse. *Intuitive Eating: A Revolutionary Anti-Diet Approach*, 4th ed. New York: St. Martin's Essentials, 2020.

Jacobsen, Maryann. *How to Raise a Mindful Eater: 8 Powerful Principles for Transforming Your Child's Relationship with Food*. San Diego: RMI Books, 2016.

Brooks, Sumner, and Amee Severson. *How to Raise an Intuitive Eater: Raising the Next Generation with Food and Body Confidence*. New York: St. Martin's Essentials, 2022.

PILLAR SIX: Food

MyPlate: myplate.gov

Siegal, Bettina Elias. *Kid Food: The Challenge of Feeding Children in a Highly Processed World*. New York: Oxford. 2019.

PILLAR SEVEN: Screens and Social Media

Common Sense Media: commonsensemedia.org

Smart Social: smartsocial.com

PILLAR EIGHT: Self-Love

The Body Positive: thebodypositive.org

Big Life Journal: biglifejournal.com

The Dove Self-Esteem Project: dove.com/us/en/dove-self-esteem
-project.html

Johnson Dias, Janice. *Parent Like It Matters: How to Raise Joyful,
Change-Making Girls.* New York: Ballantine Books, 2022.

Taylor, Sonya Renee. *The Body Is Not an Apology: The Power of Radical
Self-Love*, 2nd ed. Oakland: Berrett-Koehler Publishers, 2021.

Kite, Lindsay, and Lexie Kite. *More Than a Body: Your Body Is an
Instrument, Not an Ornament.* New York: Houghton Mifflin
Harcourt, 2021.

Gordon, Aubrey. *"You Just Need to Lose Weight": And 19 Other Myths
About Fat People.* Boston: Beacon Press, 2023.

Sole-Smith, Virginia. *Fat Talk: Parenting in the Age of Diet Culture.*
New York: Henry Holt and Co., 2023.

BOOKS FOR CHILDREN

Byers, Grace. *I Am Enough.* New York: Balzer + Bray, 2018. (For
children aged 3 to 7 years.)

Garcia, Gabi. *I Can Do Hard Things: Mindful Affirmations for Kids.*
Austin, TX: Skinned Knee Publishing, 2018. (For children aged
3 to 7 years.)

Markey, Charlotte. *Being You: The Body Image Book for Boys.* Cambridge,
UK: Cambridge University Press, 2022. (For boys aged 12+ years.)

Markey, Charlotte. *The Body Image Book for Girls: Love Yourself and
Grow Up Fearless.* Cambridge, UK: Cambridge University Press,
2020. (For girls aged 9 to 15 years.)

Taylor, Sonya Renee. *Celebrate Your Body (and It Changes, Too!): The
Ultimate Puberty Book for Girls.* Emeryville, CA: Rockridge Press,
2018. (For girls aged 8+ years.)

Kay, Katty, and Claire Shipman. *The Confidence Code for Girls: Taking Risks, Messing Up & Becoming Your Amazingly Imperfect, Totally Powerful Self.* New York: Harper Collins, 2018. (For girls aged 9 to 12 years.)

Syed, Matthew. *You Are Awesome: An Uplifting and Interactive Growth Mindset Book for Kids and Teens.* Naperville, IL: Sourcebooks Explore, 2019. (For children aged 9 to 12 years.)

ASSESSMENT
Are you Size Wise?

The following is a summary chart of the Pillars of Wellness. Use this to identify areas of progress and opportunities for improvement.

Family Culture

Learner	Striver	Thriver
• Adults criticize their own body and others'	• Self-deprecating body talk is infrequent	• No comments about bodies
• Adult or child is insecure about their body	• Adult occasionally makes comments about others	• Adult focuses on body function, not form
• Parent teases and jokes about bodies and criticizes others' habits	• Adult focuses on internal qualities of people	• Family respects all bodies
• Parent treats child with smaller or larger body differently	• Family schedules together time	• Size bias is not tolerated within or outside of the family
• Adult has few positive health behaviors (e.g., sleep, exercise, eating, etc.)	• Parent models healthful eating and enjoyment	• Child feels loved, protected, and safe
• Parent has an unaddressed history of eating and body image concerns	• Everyone in the family is treated the same	• Parent embodies a health-promoting lifestyle
• No established routines for connection (e.g., family meals or meetings)	• Improved family health habits are in progress	• Adult models health behaviors daily
• No family manifesto or mantra	• There are some family gatherings but working on more	• Family communication is prioritized
	• Family goals are being discussed (e.g., manifesto and/or mantra)	• Family has a mantra and manifesto
		• Child identifies with the family

Sleep

Learner	Striver	Thriver
• Bedtimes and wake times vary; no routine • Bedtime is chaotic • Child is rambunctious at bedtime and resists going to bed • Child is hard to wake in the morning • Child seems tired • Child sleeps in on weekends to catch up on sleep • Child gets up in the middle of the night • TV and other screens are in the bedroom • Child needs light (e.g., hallway, bedroom) to go to sleep; regularly has trouble falling asleep • Child snacks frequently after dinner; consumes caffeine-containing foods and/or beverages after lunchtime	• A sleep routine exists, but it's on and off • Calm bedtime routines, but not every night • Noise and light are minimized in the bedroom • Child is tired at the end of the day • Some technology is in the bedroom (e.g., games, phone, or computer) • Child needs a night-light to quell fear of the dark • Child gets natural sunlight most days of the week • Sometimes it's hard for child to fall asleep • Child does minimal eating after dinner; occasional late-night snack • Child occasionally drinks caffeinated beverages after midday	• Scheduled bedtimes and wake times • Child rarely resists or complains about bedtime • Calm, serene atmosphere and routines at bedtime • Sleep routine is easily re-established after vacation or breaks • Child is well-rested • Child gets morning sunlight and activity • Bedroom is tech-free • Extra light at bedtime is minimal • Child falls asleep easily • Drinks only water at bedtime • Any after-dinner snacking occurs an hour or more before bedtime • No caffeine after lunchtime

Movement

Learner	Striver	Thriver
• Child stays indoors most of the time and is highly engaged with TV and/or electronic games	• Child is signed up for sports and other activities, but inactive on down days	• Child moves every day
		• Child is engaged in a variety of physical activities, both scheduled and unscheduled
• Child relies on school or playdates for physical activities	• Parent knows child's interests and is willing to explore more	• Child gets at least an hour of physical activity daily
• Environment offers opportunities for movement, but they are not used	• Child gets outside some days of the week	• The family moves together regularly
• Parent chooses physical activities for the child	• Family engages in some physical activities together	• Child chooses physical activities, within reason
• Child may be resistant to movement	• Play space is designed for movement when indoors	• Physical activities are scheduled
• Parent may use shame and threats to motivate movement	• Parent collaborates with child in choosing physical activities	• Parent encourages fun and joyful movement
• Parent is frustrated child isn't moving more; child feels forced	• Parent is frustrated when child doesn't show motivation	• Child asks to go outside
• Child prefers sedentary activity over physical activity	• Parent focuses on fun and effort, but also on performance	• Sedentary activity is limited and adjusted to incorporate more physical movement
	• Parent avoids forcing movement	• Child is able to move as they like
	• Starting to schedule daily physical activity	

Feeding

Learner	Striver	Thriver
• Timing and location of meals and snacks are unpredictable • Parent struggles with (or doesn't enjoy) planning ahead, shopping, or cooking • Child has free access to food in the kitchen • Child snacks a lot • Meal times are chaotic • Child is pressured to eat and criticized or punished for not eating • Food rewards are used to get child to eat more or a certain food • Parent caters to the fussy eater • Parent limits second helpings and desserts • Fewer than 3 family meals per week	• Meal times are scheduled but are often delayed or changed • Parent plans meals and snacks, shops for food, and cooks frequently during the week • Parent limits access to food but feels "mean" when doing so • Child gets mixed messages about routines and access to food • Family meals take place inconsistently • Parent is mindful of how they approach feeding and is working to keep the mealtime vibe positive • Family is experimenting with self-service meals and snacks	• Predictable times and a location for meals and snacks are the norm • Parent able to recover and get back on track when life gets busy • Child understands the home food routine and established limits on food access • Child feels secure about eating • Family meals are pleasant • Parent avoids pressure to eat, catering, food restriction, and food rewards • Family gathers 3 to 5 times per week for meals • Family employs a variety of self-service and meal themes

Eating

Learner	Striver	Thriver
• Parent uses food to soothe child • Child eats due to the BLAHS • Distractions (e.g., iPad, TV, phone, books) are present at the table regularly • Child's appetite awareness is low • Parent is unsure how to respond when child is emotional about food or demonstrates impulsiveness, undereating, or overeating • Talking with child about eating is uncomfortable • Palatable foods (e.g., sweets and treats) create a struggle between parent and child • Parent is confused by child's eating behaviors and views them as intentional	• Parent aware of child's eating tendencies • Uses emotion coaching, mindful eating, and mindfulness to help child engage with appetite cues • Few distractions present when eating • Starting to teach child about appetite sensations, but this is new territory • When food triggers, temptations, and emotions exist, parent unsure how to help • Parent may be sorting through personal eating struggles • Food environment may be unsupportive for the child's eating tendencies • Avoids negative feeding dynamics	• Parent encourages mindfulness and mindful eating • No distractions present at the table • Child shows appetite awareness and follows cues of hunger and fullness • Child enjoys eating • Family has nonjudgmental dialogue about eating in the home • Child is encouraged to self-regulate eating in a variety of environments • Parent coaches child through triggers, temptations, and emotions around food • Food environment is flexible but not overly tempting to the child • Parent aims to create food enjoyment alongside an environment that doesn't invite food struggles

Food

Learner	Striver	Thriver
• Food variety is limited • Portions are larger than needed for the age of the child • Meal pattern has gaps in nutrition; child may have a deficiency • Satiating nutrients are served erratically • Minimally nutritious foods are a significant part of the eating pattern • Food shaming and guilt are used to motivate or discourage food choices • Child seems to enjoy only minimally nutritious foods • Parent worries about child's food choices • Child has limited hands-on food experiences	• Food variety is improving, but remains inconsistent • Uses filling nutrients inconsistently • Difficulty portioning favorite foods • Potential for nutrient deficits is low due to decent food variety and flexibility • Navigating minimally nutritious foods at home • Minimizes food shaming and polarizing talk about food • Connects eating enjoyment to health and well-being • Parent working on food neutrality • Child engages with food (e.g., cooking and gardening) occasionally	• Family eats a wide variety of food • Nutrient deficiency unlikely • Satiating nutrients appear at meals and snacks • Parent uses starter portions based on child's age • Parent understands nuances around food choices (e.g., food insecurity, culture, and socio-economic constraints) • No food shaming • Child enjoys most foods • Child encouraged to explore food and engage with it

Screens and Media

Learner	Striver	Thriver
• Home is chaotic • Screens are used to entertain and preoccupy the child • No formal family media use plan is in place • Child is engaged with screens each day, beyond recommended limits • Screens are in the bedroom and easy to access in the home • Parent has low awareness about media impact and intent • Family has few safety rules with media and technology • Child may be exposed to inappropriate content • Child privacy may be compromised	• Parent occasionally resorts to screens in moments of chaos • Child engages with screens beyond recommendations • Parent is beginning to put a family media plan in place • No screens in the bedroom, but they're easy to access in the home • Parent questions and discusses media content and intent with child • Some safety and controls are in place • Child is beginning to practice lateral reading and SIFT, and is gaining media literacy	• Parent schedules time for screens and digital media during the day • The home environment is calm and flows with routines • A family media plan is in place • Screen-free zones and a curfew are in place • Parent and child communicate about media engagement • Family is media literate • Child can fact-check information from media sources • Parental controls and safety rules are in place and known • Parent regularly updates media sites and programs to keep them secure

Self-Love

Learner	Striver	Thriver
• Parent is beginning to implement all the Pillars of Wellness	• Family engages with all Pillars of Wellness	• Family is practicing each Pillar of Wellness
• Parent uses each Pillar to outline goals and check progress	• Family connects self-care to self-love	• Self-care is on the weekly schedule
• Parent is becoming more engaged with self-care; considering it for child	• Parent schedules self-care time	• Self-love is a goal for each family member
• Parent is becoming more aware of size bias and stigma	• Parent encourages child to participate in self-care in a variety of ways	• Family is outspoken about body shaming and discrimination
• Parent understands societal norms around appearance are potentially dangerous for child	• Child receives positive feedback often	• Family advocates for equality, fair treatment, and dignity for all sizes
	• Parent wants to take a stand for children of all sizes	• Child is confident, loves themself, and regularly practices self-care
	• Parent is reparenting old childhood wounds and patterns	
	• Child is encouraged to self-advocate and stand up for others	

NOTES

INTRODUCTION

Today more families are raising kids with larger bodies . . . CDC. "Childhood Obesity Facts." *Overweight & Obesity.* Accessed May 17, 2022. https://www.cdc.gov/obesity/data /childhood.html.

Many children eat too many nutrient-poor foods . . . Gallagher, Siobhan. "Ultraprocessed Foods Now Comprise 2/3 of Calories in Children and Teen Diets." *Tufts Now.* August 6, 2021. https://now.tufts.edu/news-releases/ultraprocessed-foods-now-comprise-23-calories -children-and-teen-diets.

Many children eat too many nutrient-poor foods . . . Matricciani, Lisa, Catherine Paquet, Barbara Galland, Michelle A. Short, and Tim Olds. "Children's Sleep and Health: A Meta-Review." *Sleep Medicine Reviews* no. 46 (August 2019): 136–50. https://doi.org /10.1016/j.smrv.2019.04.011.

Many children eat too many nutrient-poor foods . . . CDC. "Benefits of Physical Activity for Children." Accessed June 30, 2023. https://www.cdc.gov/physicalactivity/basics/children /index.htm.

According to the Centers for Disease Control and Prevention (CDC), about 7 percent of children and teens had anxiety . . . CDC. "Anxiety and Depression in Children: Get the Facts." *Children's Mental Health.* Accessed March 8, 2023. https://www.cdc.gov /childrensmentalhealth/features/anxiety-depression-children.html.

However, during and after, rates dramatically increased with generalized anxiety at a prevalence . . . Slomski, Anita. "Pediatric Depression and Anxiety Doubled during the Pandemic." *JAMA* 326 no. 13 (October 2021): 1246. https://doi.org/10.1001 /jama.2021.16374.

And the latest statistics from the CDC . . . CDC. "CDC Report Shows Concerning Increases in Sadness and Exposure to Violence among Teen Girls and LGBQ+ Youth." *NCHHSTP Newsroom.* Accessed March 9, 2023. https://www.cdc.gov/nchhstp/newsroom/fact-sheets /healthy-youth/sadness-and-violence-among-teen-girls-and-LGBQ-youth-factsheet.html.

Children as young as three show dissatisfaction with their bodies . . . Tatangelo, Gemma, Marita P. McCabe, David Mellor, and Alex Mealey. "A Systematic Review of Body Dissatisfaction and Sociocultural Messages Related to the Body among Preschool Children." *Body Image* 18 (September 2016): 86–95. https://doi.org/10.1016/j.bodyim.2016.06.003.

By middle school, half of all girls and a third of all boys . . . National Association of Anorexia Nervosa and Associated Disorders. "Eating Disorder Statistics." *ANAD*. Accessed April 18, 2022. https://anad.org/eating-disorders-statistics/.

Over a third of parents avoid talking with their children . . . Smithers, Rebecca. "Third of Parents Fear Upsetting Children with Weight Talk, Study Finds." *The Guardian.* July 1, 2012. https://www.theguardian.com/society/2012/jul/02/parents-children -weight-talk-survey.

This number jumps to 65 percent when parents . . . Puhl, Rebecca M., Leah M. Lessard, Ellen V. Pudney, Gary D. Foster, and Michelle Cardel. "Motivations for Engaging in or Avoiding Conversations about Weight: Adolescent and Parent Perspectives." *Pediatric Obesity* 17, no 12 (December 2022): e12962. https://doi.org/10.1111/ijpo.12962.

Additionally, social determinants of health . . . Health.gov. "Social Determinants of Health." *Healthy People 2030.* Accessed December 31, 2022. https://health.gov/healthypeople /priority-areas/social-determinants-health.

For instance, there's an association between bodies with more adiposity . . . Geserick, Mandy, Mandy Vogel, Ruth Gausche, Tobias Lipek, Ulrike Spielau, E Keller, Roland Pfäffle, Wieland Kiess, and Antje Körner. "Acceleration of BMI in Early Childhood and Risk of Sustained Obesity." *The New England Journal of Medicine* 379, no. 14 (October 2018): 1303–12. https://doi.org/10.1056/nejmoa1803527.

Size reduction is not only hard to achieve . . . Mameli, Chiara, Jesse C. Krakauer, Nir Y. Krakauer, Alessandra Bosetti, Chiara Ferrari, Laura Schneider, Barbara Borsani, S. Arrigoni, Erica Pendezza, and Gian Vincenzo Zuccotti. "Effects of a Multidisciplinary Weight Loss Intervention in Overweight and Obese Children and Adolescents: 11 Years of Experience." *PLOS ONE* 12, no. 7 (July 2017): e0181095. https://doi.org/10.1371 /journal.pone.0181095.

Children who are smaller in size . . . Dobner, Jochen, and Susanne Kaser. "Body Mass Index and the Risk of Infection—from Underweight to Obesity." *Clinical Microbiology and Infection* 24, no. 1 (January 2018): 24–28. https://doi.org/10.1016/j.cmi.2017.02.013.

Embrace Size unites around fighting diet culture . . . Harrison, Christy. "What Is Diet Culture?" *Christy Harrison, MPH, RD, CEDS* (blog). Accessed August 10, 2018. https:// christyharrison.com/blog/what-is-diet-culture.

For instance, older adults (sixty-five and older) who carry extra body fat . . . Winter, Jane, Robert J. MacInnis, Naiyana Wattanapenpaiboon, and Caryl Nowson. "BMI and All-Cause Mortality in Older Adults: A Meta-Analysis." *The American Journal of Clinical Nutrition* 99, no. 4 (April 2014): 875–90. https://doi.org/10.3945/ajcn.113.068122.

Healthy lifestyle habits significantly decrease the risk of mortality . . . Matheson, Eric M., Dana E. King, and Charles J. Everett. "Healthy Lifestyle Habits and Mortality in Overweight and

Obese Individuals." *Journal of the American Board of Family Medicine* 25, no. 1 (January 2012): 9–15. https://doi.org/10.3122/jabfm.2012.01.110164.

And weight cycling . . . Lissner, Lauren, Patricia M. Odell, Ralph B. D'Agostino, Joseph Stokes, Bernard E. Kreger, Albert J. Belanger, and Kelly D. Brownell. "Variability of Body Weight and Health Outcomes in the Framingham Population." *The New England Journal of Medicine* 324, no. 26 (June 1991): 1839–44. https://doi.org/10.1056/nejm199106273242602.

Physical activity rather than weight loss . . . Gaesser, Glenn A., and Siddhartha S. Angadi. "Obesity Treatment: Weight Loss versus Increasing Fitness and Physical Activity for Reducing Health Risks." *iScience* 24, no. 10 (October 2021): 102995. https://doi.org/10.1016/j.isci.2021.102995.

And, when it comes to kids who are larger . . . van den Berg, Patricia, and Dianne Neumark-Sztainer. "Fat 'n Happy 5 Years Later: Is It Bad for Overweight Girls to Like Their Bodies?" *Journal of Adolescent Health* 41, no. 4 (October 2007): 415–17. https://doi.org/10.1016/j.jadohealth.2007.06.001.

Social media, where diet culture is pervasive . . . de Vries, Dian A., Helen Vossen, and Paulien van der Kolk–van der Boom. "Social Media and Body Dissatisfaction: Investigating the Attenuating Role of Positive Parent–Adolescent Relationships." *Journal of Youth and Adolescence* 48, no. 3 (November 2018): 527–36. https://doi.org/10.1007/s10964-018-0956-9.

THE BUILDING BLOCKS OF HEALTH

Just like your child's height . . . Geddes, Linda. "Genetic Study Homes in on Height's Heritability Mystery." *Nature* 568, no. 7753 (April 2019): 444–45. https://doi.org/10.1038/d41586-019-01157-y.

Interestingly, identical twins raised apart . . . Stunkard, Albert J., Jennifer R. Harris, Nancy L. Pedersen, and Gerald E. McClearn. "The Body-Mass Index of Twins Who Have Been Reared Apart." *The New England Journal of Medicine* 322, no. 21 (May 1990): 1483–87. https://doi.org/10.1056/nejm199005243222102.

Puberty has been occurring earlier in children . . . Farello, Giovanni, Carla Altieri, Maristella Cutini, and Gabriella Pozzobon. "Review of the Literature on Current Changes in the Timing of Pubertal Development and the Incomplete Forms of Early Puberty." *Frontiers in Pediatrics* 7 (May 2019). https://doi.org/10.3389/fped.2019.00147.

Evidence suggests girls with more body fat . . . Kaplowitz, Paul B. "Link between Body Fat and the Timing of Puberty." *Pediatrics* 121, Supplement 3 (February 2008): S208–17. https://doi.org/10.1542/peds.2007-1813f.

Early puberty might also be explained . . . Sakali, Anastasia Konstantina, Alexandra Bargiota, Ioannis G. Fatouros, Athanasios Z. Jamurtas, Djuro Macut, George Mastorakos, and Maria Papagianni. "Effects on Puberty of Nutrition-Mediated Endocrine Disruptors Employed in Agriculture." *Nutrients* 13, no. 11 (November 2021): 4184. https://doi.org/10.3390/nu13114184.

More than 4 percent of young girls experience . . . Gizem, Olgun Esin, Cetin Sirmen Kizilcan, Zeynep Şıklar, Zehra Aycan, Elif Ozsu, Ayşegül Ceran, and Merih Berberoğlu. "Investigation of Early Puberty Prevalence and Time of Addition Thelarche to Pubarche in Girls with Premature Pubarche: Two-Year Follow-up Results." *Clinical Pediatric Endocrinology* 31, no. 1 (January 2022): 25–32. https://doi.org/10.1297/cpe.2021-0042.

As such, this is the time to expose . . . Sriram, Rishi. "Why Ages 2–7 Matter So Much for Brain Development." *Edutopia*. Accessed June 24, 2020. https://www.edutopia.org /article/why-ages-2-7-matter-so-much-brain-development.

There are four stages of cognitive development . . . Mcleod, Saul. "Jean Piaget and His Theory & Stages of Cognitive Development." *SimplyPsychology*. Accessed January 24, 2024. https://www.simplypsychology.org/piaget.html.

Cognitive Developmental Stages (table) Malik, Fatima, and Raman Marwaha. "Developmental Stages of Social Emotional Development in Children." *StatPearls—NCBI Bookshelf*. Accessed April 23, 2023. http://www.ncbi.nlm.nih.gov/books/NBK534819/.

Children growing up in poverty . . . Harvard University. "Executive Function & Self-Regulation." *Center on the Developing Child*. Accessed April 21, 2022. https:// developingchild.harvard.edu/science/key-concepts/executive-function/.

Additionally, up to 40 or 50 percent . . . Masten, Ann S., and Andrew J. Barnes. "Resilience in Children: Developmental Perspectives." *Children (Basel)* 5, no. 7 (July 2018): 98. https:// doi.org/10.3390/children5070098.

Additionally, up to 40 or 50 percent . . . Seymour, Karen E., Shauna P. Reinblatt, Leora Benson, and Susan Carnell. "Overlapping Neurobehavioral Circuits in ADHD, Obesity, and Binge Eating: Evidence from Neuroimaging Research." *CNS Spectrums* 20, no. 4 (June 2015): 401–11. https://doi.org/10.1017/s1092852915000383.

Your child's social-emotional development . . . Malik, Fatima, and Raman Marwaha. "Developmental Stages of Social Emotional Development in Children." *StatPearls— NCBI Bookshelf*. Accesssed September 18, 2022. http://www.ncbi.nlm.nih.gov/books /NBK534819/.

Temperament is something your child is born with . . . Malik, Fatima, and Raman Marwaha. "Developmental Stages of Social Emotional Development in Children." *StatPearls— NCBI Bookshelf*. Accessed September 18, 2022. http://www.ncbi.nlm.nih.gov/books /NBK534819/.

Children need approval . . . Harter, Susan. *The Construction of the Self: A Developmental Perspective*. New York: Guilford Press, 1999.

But the opposite—criticism, low acceptance . . . Garber, Judy, and Cynthia Flynn. "Predictors of Depressive Cognitions in Young Adolescents." *Cognitive Therapy and Research* 25, no. 4 (August 2001): 353–76. https://doi.org/10.1023/a:1005530402239.

Homes with warm and responsive parents . . . Orth, Ulrich. "The Family Environment in Early Childhood Has a Long-Term Effect on Self-Esteem: A Longitudinal Study from Birth to Age 27 Years." *Journal of Personality and Social Psychology* 114, no. 4 (April 2018): 637–55. https://doi.org/10.1037/pspp0000143.

Hypertension is more common in children . . . Cuda, Suzanne, and Marisa Censani. "Pediatric Obesity Algorithm: A Practical Approach to Obesity Diagnosis and Management." *Frontiers in Pediatrics* 6 (January 2019). https://doi.org/10.3389/fped.2018.00431.

Seven percent of US kids have high cholesterol . . . CDC. "High Cholesterol Facts." *Cholesterol.* Accessed May 15, 2023. https://www.cdc.gov/cholesterol/facts.htm.

Pediatricians routinely check blood cholesterol . . . HealthyChildren.org. "Cholesterol Levels in Children and Adolescents." Accessed August 20, 2020. https://www.healthychildren.org /english/healthy-living/nutrition/pages/cholesterol-levels-in-children-and-adolescents.aspx.

The prevalence of both types of diabetes . . . Lawrence, Jean M., Jasmin Divers, Scott Isom, Sharon Saydah, Giuseppina Imperatore, Catherine Pihoker, Santica M. Marcovina, et al. "Trends in Prevalence of Type 1 and Type 2 Diabetes in Children and Adolescents in the US, 2001–2017." *JAMA* 326, no. 8 (August 2021): 717–27. https://doi.org/10.1001 /jama.2021.11165.

Studies show that vitamin D . . . Fiamenghi, Verônica Indicatti, and Elza Daniel de Mello. "Vitamin D Deficiency in Children and Adolescents with Obesity: A Meta-Analysis." *Jornal de Pediatria* 97, no. 3 (May–June 2021): 273–79. https://doi.org/10.1016/j.jped .2020.08.006.

Studies show a 25 percent increased risk of arm and leg fractures . . . Fintini, Danilo, Stefano Cianfarani, Marta Cofini, A Andreoletti, Graziamaria Ubertini, Marco Cappa, and Melania Manco. "The Bones of Children with Obesity." *Frontiers in Endocrinology* no. 11 (April 2020). https://doi.org/10.3389/fendo.2020.00200.

Smaller children may have . . . Bialo, Shara R., and Catherine M. Gordon. "Underweight, Overweight, and Pediatric Bone Fragility: Impact and Management." *Current Osteoporosis Reports* 12, no. 3 (July 2014): 319–28. https://doi.org/10.1007/s11914-014-0226-z.

Children who have more body fat . . . Singendonk, Maartje, Eline Goudswaard, Miranda Langendam, Michiel P. van Wijk, Faridi S. van Etten-Jamaludin, Marc A. Benninga, and Merit M. Tabbers. "Prevalence of Gastroesophageal Reflux Disease Symptoms in Infants and Children: A Systematic Review." *Journal of Pediatric Gastroenterology and Nutrition* 68, no. 6 (June 2019): 811–17. https://doi.org/10.1097/mpg.0000000000002280.

Studies show that children who experience size discrimination . . . Guardabassi, Veronica, Alberto Mirisola, and Carlo Tomasetto. "How Is Weight Stigma Related to Children's Health-Related Quality of Life? A Model Comparison Approach." *Quality of Life Research* 27, no. 1 (September 2017): 173–83. https://doi.org/10.1007/s11136-017-1701-7.

In children with larger bodies . . . Puhl, Rebecca M., and Leah M. Lessard. "Weight Stigma in Youth: Prevalence, Consequences, and Considerations for Clinical Practice." *Current Obesity Reports* 9, no. 4 (October 2020): 402–11. https://doi.org/10.1007 /s13679-020-00408-8.

Furthermore, children and teens . . . Puhl, Rebecca M., Melanie M. Wall, Chen Chen, S. Bryn Austin, Marla E. Eisenberg, and Dianne Neumark-Sztainer. "Experiences of Weight Teasing in Adolescence and Weight-Related Outcomes in Adulthood: A 15-Year Longitudinal Study." *Preventive Medicine* 100 (July 2017): 173–79. https://doi .org/10.1016/j.ypmed.2017.04.023.

Bullying and teasing . . . Puhl, Rebecca M., and Leah M. Lessard. "Weight Stigma in Youth: Prevalence, Consequences, and Considerations for Clinical Practice." *Current Obesity Reports* 9, no. 4 (October 2020): 402–11. https://doi.org/10.1007/s13679-020-00408-8.

Unfortunately, size stigma happens . . . Palad, Carl J., Siddharth Yarlagadda, and Fatima Cody Stanford. "Weight Stigma and Its Impact on Paediatric Care." *Current Opinion in Endocrinology, Diabetes and Obesity* 26, no. 1 (February 2019): 19–24. https://doi.org /10.1097/med.0000000000000453.

Even doctors, nurses, and other health-care providers . . . Puhl, Rebecca M., and Leah M. Lessard. "Weight Stigma in Youth: Prevalence, Consequences, and Considerations for Clinical Practice." *Current Obesity Reports* 9, no. 4 (October 2020): 402–11. https://doi .org/10.1007/s13679-020-00408-8.

Feeling unhappy about one's size . . . Dion, Jacinthe, Jennifer Hains, Patrick Vachon, Jacques Plouffe, Luc Laberge, Michel Perron, Pierre McDuff, Émilia Kalinova, and Mario Leone. "Correlates of Body Dissatisfaction in Children." *The Journal of Pediatrics* 171 (April 2016): 202–7. https://doi.org/10.1016/j.jpeds.2015.12.045.

Thankfully, scientists have teased out the factors . . . Masten, Ann S., and Andrew J. Barnes. "Resilience in Children: Developmental Perspectives." *Children (Basel)* 5, no. 7 (July 2018): 98. https://doi.org/10.3390/children5070098.

PILLAR ONE

Strong family bonds . . . Wilcox, Brad, and Hal Boyd. "The Nuclear Family Is Still Indispensable." *The Atlantic.* February 21, 2020. https://www.theatlantic.com/ideas /archive/2020/02/nuclear-family-still-indispensable/606841/.

In fact, for a child, the cornerstone to thriving . . . Whitaker, Robert C., Tracy Dearth-Wesley, Allison N. Herman, Anne-Sophie van Wingerden, and Delaine W. Winn. "Family Connection and Flourishing among Adolescents in 26 Countries." *Pediatrics* 149, no. 6 (June 2022): e2021055263. https://doi.org/10.1542/peds.2021-055263.

Children who have the greatest family connectedness . . . Whitaker, Robert C., Tracy Dearth-Wesley, Allison N. Herman, Anne-Sophie van Wingerden, and Delaine W. Winn. "Family Connection and Flourishing among Adolescents in 26 Countries." *Pediatrics* 149, no. 6 (June 2022): e2021055263. https://doi.org/10.1542/peds.2021-055263.

The opposite—loose family ties . . . Campos, Belinda, Jodie B. Ullman, Adrian Aguilera, and Christine Dunkel Schetter. "Familism and Psychological Health: The Intervening Role of Closeness and Social Support." *Cultural Diversity & Ethnic Minority Psychology* 20, no. 2 (April 2014): 191–201. https://doi.org/10.1037/a0034094.

Parents with healthful behaviors . . . Coto, Jennifer, Elizabeth R. Pulgaron, Paulo A. Graziano, Daniel M. Bagner, Manuela Villa, Jamil A. Malik, and Alan M. Delamater. "Parents as Role Models: Associations between Parent and Young Children's Weight, Dietary Intake, and Physical Activity in a Minority Sample." *Maternal and Child Health Journal* 23, no. 7 (July 2019): 943–50. https://doi.org/10.1007/s10995-018-02722-z.

Ironically, what a parent eats is less *important* . . . Vaughn, Amber, Chantel L. Martin, and Dianne S. Ward. "What Matters Most—What Parents Model or What Parents Eat?" *Appetite* 126 (July 2018): 102–7. https://doi.org/10.1016/j.appet.2018.03.025.

And when you demonstrate enjoyment . . . Yee, Andrew, May O. Lwin, and Shirley S. Ho. "The Influence of Parental Practices on Child Promotive and Preventive Food Consumption Behaviors: A Systematic Review and Meta-Analysis." *International Journal of Behavioral Nutrition and Physical Activity* 14, no. 47 (April 2017) https://doi.org/10.1186/s12966-017-0501-3.

Family meals are the most influential . . . Mahmood, Lubna, Paloma Flores-Barrantes, Luis A. Moreno, Yannis Manios, and Esther M. Gonzalez-Gil. "The Influence of Parental Dietary Behaviors and Practices on Children's Eating Habits." *Nutrients* 13, no. 4 (April 2021): 1138. https://doi.org/10.3390/nu13041138.

And if you cut the time spent . . . Xu, Huilan, Li Ming Wen, and Chris Rissel. "Associations of Parental Influences with Physical Activity and Screen Time among Young Children: A Systematic Review." *Journal of Obesity* 2015 (January 2015): 1–23. https://doi.org/10.1155/2015/546925.

Parents of children who have . . . Lydecker, Janet A., Elizabeth O'Brien, and Carlos M. Grilo. "Parents Have Both Implicit and Explicit Biases against Children with Obesity." *Journal of Behavioral Medicine* 41, no. 6 (May 2018): 784–91. https://doi.org/10.1007/s10865-018-9929-4.

For children, size discrimination . . . Pont, Stephen J., Rebecca M. Puhl, Stephen Cook, Wendelin Slusser. "Stigma Experienced by Children and Adolescents with Obesity." *Pediatrics* 140, no. 6 (December 2017): e20173034. https://doi.org/10.1542/peds.2017-3034.

Children as young as three years old . . . Skinner, Asheley Cockrell, Keith Payne, Andrew J. Perrin, A. T. Panter, Janna Howard, Anna M. Bardone-Cone, Cynthia M. Bulik, Michael Steiner, and Eliana M. Perrin. "Implicit Weight Bias in Children Age 9 to 11 Years." *Pediatrics* 140, no. 1 (July 2017): e20163936. https://doi.org/10.1542/peds.2016-3936.

Sadly, 37 percent of teenagers . . . Puhl, Rebecca M., Jamie Lee Peterson, and Joerg Luedicke. "Weight-Based Victimization: Bullying Experiences of Weight Loss Treatment–Seeking Youth." *Pediatrics* 131, no. 1 (January 2013): e1–9. https://doi.org/10.1542/peds.2012-1106.

Women in larger bodies recalled . . . Puhl, Rebecca M., and Kelly D. Brownell. "Confronting and Coping with Weight Stigma: An Investigation of Overweight and Obese Adults." *Obesity* 14, no. 10 (September 2012): 1802–15. https://doi.org/10.1038/oby.2006.208.

However, a negative *family culture* . . . Lazarevic, Vanja, Flavia Crovetto, Alyson F. Shapiro, and Stephanie Nguyen. "Family Dynamics Moderate the Impact of Discrimination on Wellbeing for Latino Young Adults." *Cultural Diversity & Ethnic Minority Psychology* 27, no. 2 (April 2021): 214–26. https://doi.org/10.1037/cdp0000344.

Studies show that children whose mothers . . . Martini, Maria Giulia, Manuela Barona-Martinez, and Nadia Micali. "Eating Disorders Mothers and Their Children: A Systematic Review of the Literature." *Archives of Women's Mental Health* 23, no. 4 (January 2020): 449–67. https://doi.org/10.1007/s00737-020-01019-x.

Protective factors include . . . Langdon-Daly, Jasmin, and Lucy Serpell. "Protective Factors against Disordered Eating in Family Systems: A Systematic Review of Research." *Journal of Eating Disorders* 5, no. 12 (March 2017). https://doi.org/10.1186/s40337-017-0141-7.

Importantly, when parents and extended family . . . Langdon-Daly, Jasmin, and Lucy Serpell. "Protective Factors against Disordered Eating in Family Systems: A Systematic Review of Research." *Journal of Eating Disorders* 5, no. 12 (March 2017). https://doi.org/10.1186/s40337-017-0141-7.

Dieting and especially talking about food . . . Balantekin, Katherine N. "The Influence of Parental Dieting Behavior on Child Dieting Behavior and Weight Status." *Current Obesity Reports* 8, no. 2 (March 2019): 137–44. https://doi.org/10.1007/s13679-019-00338-0.

Instead of focusing on shortcomings . . . Neff, Kristin. "What Self-Compassion Is and the Three Elements of Self-Compassion." *Self-Compassion* (blog). Accessed June 7, 2022. https://self-compassion.org/the-three-elements-of-self-compassion-2/.

PILLAR TWO

Nearly half of US kids . . . American Academy of Pediatrics. "Only Half of US Children Get Enough Sleep During the Week." *ScienceDaily.* October 25, 2019. http://www.sciencedaily.com/releases/2019/10/191025075604.htm.

Age-Based Sleep Recommendations for Children (table) Paruthi, Shalini, Lee J. Brooks, Carolyn D'Ambrosio, Wendy A. Hall, Suresh Kotagal, Robin M. Lloyd, Beth A. Malow, et al. "Consensus Statement of the American Academy of Sleep Medicine on the Recommended Amount of Sleep for Healthy Children: Methodology and Discussion." *Journal of Clinical Sleep Medicine* 12, no. 11 (November 2016): 1549–61. https://doi.org/10.5664/jcsm.6288.

The American Academy of Pediatrics . . . Au, Rhoda, Mary A. Carskadon, Richard P. Millman, Amy R. Wolfson, Paula K. Braverman, William P. Adelman, Cora Collette Breuner, et al. "School Start Times for Adolescents." *Pediatrics* 134, no. 3 (September 2014): 642–49. https://doi.org/10.1542/peds.2014-1697.

Short-term use is considered safe . . . HealthyChildren.Org. "Melatonin for Kids: What Parents Should Know About This Sleep Aid." Accessed April 27, 2023. https://www.healthychildren.org/English/healthy-living/sleep/Pages/melatonin-and-childrens-sleep.aspx.

The National Sleep Foundation and other experts . . . Ohayon, Maurice M., Emerson M. Wickwire, Max Hirshkowitz, Steven M. Albert, Alon Y. Avidan, Frank J. Daly, Yves Dauvilliers, et al. "National Sleep Foundation's Sleep Quality Recommendations: First Report." *Sleep Health* 3, no. 1 (February 2017): 6–19. https://doi.org/10.1016/j.sleh.2016.11.006.

The National Sleep Foundation and other experts . . . Phillips, Shameka, Ann Hammack Johnson, Maria R. Shirey, and Marti Rice. "Sleep Quality in School-Aged Children: A Concept Analysis." *Journal of Pediatric Nursing* 52 (May 2020): 54–63. https://doi.org/10.1016/j.pedn.2020.02.043.

About 70 percent of preteens and teens . . . CDC. "Sleep in Middle and High School Students." *Healthy Schools.* Accessed September 10, 2020. https://www.cdc.gov/healthyschools /features/students-sleep.htm.

For example, children who get adequate sleep . . . Chaput, Jean-Philippe, Casey Gray, Veronica J. Poitras, Valerie Carson, Reut Gruber, Tim Olds, Shelly K. Weiss, et al. "Systematic Review of the Relationships between Sleep Duration and Health Indicators in School-Aged Children and Youth." *Applied Physiology, Nutrition, and Metabolism* 41, no. 6, Supplement 3 (June 2016): S266–82. https://doi.org/10.1139/apnm-2015-0627.

Children with longer sleep duration . . . Matricciani, Lisa, Catherine Paquet, Barbara Galland, Michelle A. Short, and Tim Olds. "Children's Sleep and Health: A Meta-Review." *Sleep Medicine Reviews* 46 (August 2019): 136–50. https://doi.org/10.1016/j.smrv.2019.04.011.

Lack of sleep may disturb emotional . . . Tempesta, Daniela, Valentina Socci, Luigi De Gennaro, and Michele Ferrara. "Sleep and Emotional Processing." *Sleep Medicine Reviews* 40 (August 2018): 183–95. https://doi.org/10.1016/j.smrv.2017.12.005.

Inadequate sleep may make them more anxious . . . Palmer, Cara A., and Candice A. Alfano. "Anxiety Modifies the Emotional Effects of Sleep Loss." *Current Opinion in Psychology* 34 (August 2020): 100–104. https://doi.org/10.1016/j.copsyc.2019.12.001.

In a study of three- to ten-year-olds . . . Sundell, Anna Lena, and Charlotte Angelhoff. "Sleep and Its Relation to Health-Related Quality of Life in 3–10-Year-Old Children." *BMC Public Health* 21, no. 1 (June 2021). https://doi.org/10.1186/s12889-021-11038-7.

Longitudinal studies . . . Chaput, Jean-Philippe, Casey Gray, Veronica J. Poitras, Valerie Carson, Reut Gruber, Tim Olds, Shelly K. Weiss, et al. "Systematic Review of the Relationships between Sleep Duration and Health Indicators in School-Aged Children and Youth." *Applied Physiology, Nutrition, and Metabolism* 41, no. 6, Supplement 3 (June 2016): S266–82. https://doi.org/10.1139/apnm-2015-0627.

Longitudinal studies . . . Wheaton, Anne G., and Angelika H. Claussen. "Short Sleep Duration among Infants, Children, and Adolescents Aged 4 Months–17 Years—United States, 2016–2018." *Morbidity and Mortality Weekly Report* 70, no. 38 (September 2021): 1315–21. https://doi.org/10.15585/mmwr.mm7038a1.

Additionally, between birth and four years . . . Chaput, Jean-Philippe, Casey Gray, Veronica J. Poitras, Valerie Carson, Reut Gruber, Catherine S. Birken, Joanna E. MacLean, Salomé Aubert, Margaret Sampson, and Mark S. Tremblay. "Systematic Review of the Relationships between Sleep Duration and Health Indicators in the Early Years (0–4 Years)." *BMC Public Health* 17, Supplement 5 (November 2017). https://doi.org/10.1186 /s12889-017-4850-2.

Overall, research suggests that a shorter duration . . . Wheaton, Anne G., and Angelika H. Claussen. "Short Sleep Duration among Infants, Children, and Adolescents Aged 4 Months–17 Years—United States, 2016–2018." *Morbidity and Mortality Weekly Report* 70, no. 38 (September 2021): 1315–21. https://doi.org/10.15585/mmwr.mm7038a1.

Some research suggests that every additional hour . . . Miller, Michelle A., Marlot Kruisbrink, J. Wallace, Chen Ji, and Francesco P. Cappuccio. "Sleep Duration and Incidence of Obesity in Infants, Children, and Adolescents: A Systematic Review and Meta-Analysis of Prospective Studies." *Sleep* 41, no. 4 (April 2018): zsy018. https://doi.org/10.1093 /sleep/zsy018.

When sleep-wake patterns are disturbed . . . Narang, Indra, and Joseph L Mathew. "Childhood Obesity and Obstructive Sleep Apnea." *Journal of Nutrition and Metabolism* 2012 (January 2012): 1–8. https://doi.org/10.1155/2012/134202.

Interestingly, poor sleep may change . . . St-Onge, Marie-Pierre, Andrew McReynolds, Zalak B. Trivedi, Amy L. Roberts, Melissa Sy, and Joy Hirsch. "Sleep Restriction Leads to Increased Activation of Brain Regions Sensitive to Food Stimuli." *The American Journal of Clinical Nutrition* 95, no. 4 (April 2012): 818–24. https://doi.org/10.3945/ajcn.111.027383.

Specifically, they ate . . . Mullins, Elsa N., Alison L. Miller, Sherin S. Cherian, Julie C. Lumeng, Kenneth P. Wright, Salome Kurth, and Monique K. LeBourgeois. "Acute Sleep Restriction Increases Dietary Intake in Preschool-Age Children." *Journal of Sleep Research* 26, no. 1 (February 2017): 48–54. https://doi.org/10.1111/jsr.12450.

When looking at sleep as an influence . . . Matricciani, Lisa, Dorothea Dumuid, Catherine Paquet, François Fraysse, Yichao Wang, Louise A. Baur, Markus Juonala, et al. "Sleep and Cardiometabolic Health in Children and Adults: Examining Sleep as a Component of the 24-h Day." *Sleep Medicine* 78 (February 2021): 63–74. https://doi.org/10.1016 /j.sleep.2020.12.001.

In fact, a third of children . . . Wheaton, Anne G., and Angelika H. Claussen. "Short Sleep Duration among Infants, Children, and Adolescents Aged 4 Months–17 Years—United States, 2016–2018." *Morbidity and Mortality Weekly Report* 70, no. 38 (September 2021): 1315–21. https://doi.org/10.15585/mmwr.mm7038a1.

Two-thirds of middle schoolers . . . CDC. "Sleep in Middle and High School Students." *Healthy Schools*. Accessed September 10, 2020. https://www.cdc.gov/healthyschools /features/students-sleep.htm.

But as kids get older . . . Lewien, Christiane, Jon Genuneit, Christof Meigen, Wieland Kiess, and Tanja Poulain. "Sleep-Related Difficulties in Healthy Children and Adolescents." *BMC Pediatrics* 21, no. 1 (February 2021). https://doi.org/10.1186/s12887-021-02529-y.

The light coming from screens . . . Fadzil, Ammar. "Factors Affecting the Quality of Sleep in Children." *Children (Basel)* 8, no. 2 (Feburary 2021): 122. https://doi.org/10.3390 /children8020122.

One study found that children . . . Singh, Gopal K., and Mary Kay Kenney. "Rising Prevalence and Neighborhood, Social, and Behavioral Determinants of Sleep Problems in US Children and Adolescents, 2003–2012." *Sleep Disorders* 2013 (January 2013): 1–15. https://doi.org/10.1155/2013/394320.

A third of children who report sleep problems . . . Kolip, Petra, Ronny Kuhnert, and Anke-Christine Saß. "Social, Health-Related, and Environmental Factors Influencing Sleep Problems of Children, Adolescents and Young Adults." *PubMed* 7, Supplement 2 (June 2022): 2–19. https://doi.org/10.25646/9879.

About 2–3 percent of children . . . Lo Bue, Anna, Adriana Salvaggio, and Giuseppe Insalaco. "Obstructive Sleep Apnea in Developmental Age: A Narrative Review." *European*

Journal of Pediatrics 179, no. 3 (January 2020): 357–65. https://doi.org/10.1007/s00431-019-03557-8.

Obstructive sleep apnea is increasingly . . . Lo Bue, Anna, Adriana Salvaggio, and Giuseppe Insalaco. "Obstructive Sleep Apnea in Developmental Age: A Narrative Review." *European Journal of Pediatrics* 179, no. 3 (January 2020): 357–65. https://doi.org/10.1007/s00431-019-03557-8.

Children with larger bodies . . . Narang, Indra, and Joseph L. Mathew. "Childhood Obesity and Obstructive Sleep Apnea." *Journal of Nutrition and Metabolism* 2012 (January 2020): 1–8. https://doi.org/10.1155/2012/134202.

Currently, the incidence of OSA . . . Andersen, Ida Gillberg, Jens Christian Holm, and Preben Homøe. "Obstructive Sleep Apnea in Obese Children and Adolescents, Treatment Methods and Outcome of Treatment—A Systematic Review." *International Journal of Pediatric Otorhinolaryngology* 87 (August 2016): 190–97. https://doi.org/10.1016/j.ijporl.2016.06.017.

A recent study found that smaller kids . . . Johnson, Courtney, Taylor Leavitt, Shiva Daram, Romaine F. Johnson, and Ron B. Mitchell. "Obstructive Sleep Apnea in Underweight Children." *Otolaryngology-Head and Neck Surgery* 167, no. 7 (November 2021): 566–72. https://doi.org/10.1177/01945998211058722.

It's recommended that children younger than twelve years . . . AACAP. "Caffeine and Children." American Academy of Child & Adolescent Psychiatry. Accessed August 22, 2022. https://www.aacap.org/AACAP/Families_and_Youth/Facts_for_Families/FFF-Guide/Caffeine_and_Children-131.aspx.

Yet 73 percent . . . Branum, Amy M., Lauren M. Rossen, and Kenneth C. Schoendorf. "Trends in Caffeine Intake Among US Children and Adolescents." *Pediatrics* 133, no. 3 (March 2014): 386–93. https://doi.org/10.1542/peds.2013-2877.

Foods such as milk products . . . St-Onge, Marie-Pierre, Anja Mikic, and Cara E Pietrolungo. "Effects of Diet on Sleep Quality." *Advances in Nutrition* 7, no. 5 (September 2016): 938–49. https://doi.org/10.3945/an.116.012336.

PILLAR THREE

Physical activity builds muscle . . . US Department of Health and Human Services. *Physical Activity Guidelines for Americans, 2nd edition.* Accessed November 1, 2022. https://health.gov/sites/default/files/2019-09/Physical_Activity_Guidelines_2nd_edition.pdf.

Children who are larger . . . Gaesser, Glenn A., and Siddhartha S. Angadi. "Obesity Treatment: Weight Loss versus Increasing Fitness and Physical Activity for Reducing Health Risks." *iScience* 24, no. 10 (October 2021): 102995. https://doi.org/10.1016/j.isci.2021.102995.

Physical activity and exercise . . . Dimitri, Paul, Kush Joshi, and Natasha Jones. "Moving More: Physical Activity and Its Positive Effects on Long Term Conditions in Children and Young People." *Archives of Disease in Childhood* 105, no. 11 (November 2020): 1035–40. https://doi.org/10.1136/archdischild-2019-318017.

Children and adults spend . . . Katzmarzyk, Peter T., Kenneth E. Powell, John M. Jakicic, Richard P. Troiano, Katrina L. Piercy, and Bethany Tennant. "Sedentary Behavior and Health: Update from the 2018 Physical Activity Guidelines Advisory Committee." *Medicine and Science in Sports and Exercise* 51, no. 6 (June 2019): 1227–41. https://doi .org/10.1249/mss.0000000000001935.

During the COVID-19 pandemic . . . Dunton, Genevieve F., Bridgette Do, and Shirlene Wang. "Early Effects of the COVID-19 Pandemic on Physical Activity and Sedentary Behavior in Children Living in the U.S." *BMC Public Health* 20, no. 1 (September 2020). https://doi.org/10.1186/s12889-020-09429-3.

Children aged six years and older . . . US Department of Health and Human Services. *Physical Activity Guidelines for Americans, 2nd edition.* https://health.gov/sites/default/files/2019-09 /Physical_Activity_Guidelines_2nd_edition.pdf.

Goals for Physical Activity (table) Raghuveer, Geetha, Jacob Hartz, David R. Lubans, T. Takken, Jennifer L. Wiltz, Michele Mietus-Snyder, Amanda M. Perak, Connie U. Smith, Nicholas Pietris, and Nicholas M. Edwards. "Cardiorespiratory Fitness in Youth: An Important Marker of Health: A Scientific Statement from the American Heart Association." *Circulation* 147, no. 7 (July 2020): e101–e118. https://doi.org/10.1161 /cir.0000000000000866.

For instance, children with a chronic condition . . . CDC. "Benefits of Physical Activity for Children." Accessed October 16, 2023. https://www.cdc.gov/physicalactivity/basics /index.htm.

Some of the latest statistics indicate . . . Gray, Casey, Rebecca E. Gibbons, Richard Larouche, Ellen Beate Hansen Sandseter, Adam Bienenstock, Mariana Brussoni, Guylaine Chabot, et al. "What Is the Relationship between Outdoor Time and Physical Activity, Sedentary Behaviour, and Physical Fitness in Children? A Systematic Review." *International Journal of Environmental Research and Public Health* 12, no. 6 (June 2015): 6455–74. https://doi .org/10.3390/ijerph120606455.

Yet time outdoors has been linked to . . . Gray, Casey, Rebecca E. Gibbons, Richard Larouche, Ellen Beate Hansen Sandseter, Adam Bienenstock, Mariana Brussoni, Guylaine Chabot, et al. "What Is the Relationship between Outdoor Time and Physical Activity, Sedentary Behaviour, and Physical Fitness in Children? A Systematic Review." *International Journal of Environmental Research and Public Health* 12, no. 6 (June 2015): 6455–74. https://doi .org/10.3390/ijerph120606455.

The bad news is if you aren't active . . . Gerards, Sanne M. P. L., Dave H. H. Van Kann, Stef Kremers, Maria Jansen, and Jessica S. Gubbels. "Do Parenting Practices Moderate the Association between the Physical Neighbourhood Environment and Changes in Children's Time Spent at Various Physical Activity Levels? An Exploratory Longitudinal Study." *BMC Public Health* 21, no. 1 (January 2021): 68. https://doi.org/10.1186 /s12889-021-10224-x.

And when you support what is needed . . . Gerards, Sanne M. P. L., Dave H. H. Van Kann, Stef Kremers, Maria Jansen, and Jessica S. Gubbels. "Do Parenting Practices Moderate the Association between the Physical Neighbourhood Environment and Changes in Children's Time Spent at Various Physical Activity Levels? An Exploratory Longitudinal

Study." *BMC Public Health* 21, no. 1 (January 2021): 68. https://doi.org/10.1186 /s12889-021-10224-x.

In fact, these opportunities have been steadily declining . . . Weaver, R. Glenn, Rafael Miranda Tassitano, Maria Cecília Marinho Tenório, Keith Brazendale, and Michael W. Beets. "Temporal Trends in Children's School Day Moderate to Vigorous Physical Activity: A Systematic Review and Meta-Regression Analysis." *Journal of Physical Activity & Health* 18, no. 11 (October 2021): 1446–67. https://doi.org/10.1123/jpah.2021-0254.

Additionally, the actual *physical activity* . . . Demetriou, Yolanda, Anne Reimers, Marianna Alesi, Lidia Scifo, Carla Chicau Borrego, Diogo Monteiro, and Anne Kelso. "Effects of School-Based Interventions on Motivation towards Physical Activity in Children and Adolescents: Protocol for a Systematic Review." *Systematic Reviews* 8, no. 1 (May 2019): 113. https://doi.org/10.1186/s13643-019-1029-1.

Children cut their usual steps . . . Grimes, Amanda, Joseph S. Lightner, Katlyn Eighmy, Chelsea Steel, Robin P. Shook, and Jordan Carlson. "Decreased Physical Activity among Youth Resulting from COVID-19 Pandemic–Related School Closures: Natural Experimental Study." *JMIR Formative Research* 6, no. 4 (April 2022): e35854. https:// doi.org/10.2196/35854.

Physical activity dropped significantly . . . Paterson, Derek C, Katelynn Ramage, Sarah A. Moore, Negin Riazi, Mark S. Tremblay, and Guy Faulkner. "Exploring the Impact of COVID-19 on the Movement Behaviors of Children and Youth: A Scoping Review of Evidence after the First Year." *Journal of Sport and Health Science* 10, no. 6 (December 2021): 675–89. https://doi.org/10.1016/j.jshs.2021.07.001.

Size and exercise assumptions aside . . . Kelley, George A., Kristi S. Kelley, and Russell R. Pate. "Exercise and Adiposity in Overweight and Obese Children and Adolescents: A Systematic Review with Network Meta-Analysis of Randomised Trials." *BMJ Open* 9, no. 11 (November 2019): e031220. https://doi.org/10.1136/bmjopen-2019-031220.

A focus on fitness also skirts . . . Gaesser, Glenn A., and Siddhartha S. Angadi. "Obesity Treatment: Weight Loss versus Increasing Fitness and Physical Activity for Reducing Health Risks." *iScience* 24, no. 10 (September 2021): 102995. https://doi.org/10.1016 /j.isci.2021.102995.

Improving cardiorespiratory fitness . . . Raghuveer, Geetha, Jacob Hartz, David R. Lubans, T. Takken, Jennifer L. Wiltz, Michele Mietus-Snyder, Amanda M. Perak, Connie U. Smith, Nicholas Pietris, and Nicholas M. Edwards. "Cardiorespiratory Fitness in Youth: An Important Marker of Health: A Scientific Statement from the American Heart Association." *Circulation* 142, no. 7 (August 2020): e101–e118. https://doi.org/10.1161 /cir.0000000000000866.

Even children with chronic health conditions . . . Dimitri, Paul, Kush Joshi, and Natasha Jones. "Moving More: Physical Activity and Its Positive Effects on Long Term Conditions in Children and Young People." *Archives of Disease in Childhood* 105, no. 11 (November 2020): 1035–40. https://doi.org/10.1136/archdischild-2019-318017.

A study of seven- and eight-year-olds . . . Lohbeck, Annette, Philipp Von Keitz, Andreas Hohmann, and Monika Daseking. "Children's Physical Self-Concept, Motivation, and Physical Performance: Does Physical Self-Concept or Motivation Play a Mediating Role?" *Frontiers in Psychology* 12 (April 2021). https://doi.org/10.3389/fpsyg.2021.669936.

Furthermore, being with friends or family . . . Mema, Ensela, Everett S. Spain, Corby K. Martin, James O. Hill, R. Drew Sayer, Howard D. McInvale, Lee A. Evans, Nicholas H. Gist, Alexander D. Borowsky, and Diana M. Thomas. "Social Influences on Physical Activity for Establishing Criteria Leading to Exercise Persistence." *PLOS ONE* 17, no. 10 (October 2022): e0274259. https://doi.org/10.1371/journal.pone.0274259.

When we focus on performance outcomes . . . Demetriou, Yolanda, Anne Reimers, Marianna Alesi, Lidia Scifo, Carla Chicau Borrego, Diogo Monteiro, and Anne Kelso. "Effects of School-Based Interventions on Motivation towards Physical Activity in Children and Adolescents: Protocol for a Systematic Review." *Systematic Reviews* 8, no. 1 (May 2019). https://doi.org/10.1186/s13643-019-1029-1.

PILLAR FOUR

This is called intergenerational feeding . . . Lev-Ari, Lilac, Ada H. Zohar, Rachel Bachner-Melman, and Auriane Totah Hanhart. "Intergenerational Transmission of Child Feeding Practices." *International Journal of Environmental Research and Public Health* 18, no. 15 (August 2021): 8183. https://doi.org/10.3390/ijerph18158183.

Overriding fullness cues by feeding more . . . Schneider-Worthington, Camille R., Paige K. Berger, Michael I. Goran, and Sarah-Jeanne Salvy. "Learning to Overeat in Infancy: Concurrent and Prospective Relationships between Maternal BMI, Feeding Practices, and Child Eating Response among Hispanic Mothers and Children." *Pediatric Obesity* 16, no. 6 (November 2020): e12756. https://doi.org/10.1111/ijpo.12756.

Currently there are . . . Lopez, Nanette V., Susan M. Schembre, Britni R. Belcher, Sydney O'Connor, Jaclyn P. Maher, Reout Arbel, Gayla Margolin, and Genevieve F. Dunton. "Parenting Styles, Food-Related Parenting Practices, and Children's Healthy Eating: A Mediation Analysis to Examine Relationships between Parenting and Child Diet." *Appetite* 128 (September 2018): 205–13. https://doi.org/10.1016/j.appet.2018.06.021.

The controlling feeding style . . . Vaughn, Amber, Dianne S. Ward, Jennifer O. Fisher, Myles S. Faith, Sheryl O. Hughes, Stef Kremers, Dara R. Musher-Eizenman, Teresia M. O'Connor, Heather Patrick, and Thomas G. Power. "Fundamental Constructs in Food Parenting Practices: A Content Map to Guide Future Research." *Nutrition Reviews* 74, no. 2 (February 2016): 98–117. https://doi.org/10.1093/nutrit/nuv061.

If you have a child with a larger body . . . Power, Thomas G., Ashley E. Beck, Jennifer O. Fisher, Nilda Micheli, Teresia M. O'Connor, and Sheryl O. Hughes. "Observations of Maternal Feeding Practices and Styles and Young Children's Obesity Risk: A Longitudinal Study of Hispanic Mothers with Low Incomes." *Childhood Obesity* 17, no. 1 (January 2021): 16–25. https://doi.org/10.1089/chi.2020.0178.

If you have a child with a larger body . . . Russell, Catherine Georgina, Jillian J. Haszard, Rachael W Taylor, Anne-Louise M Heath, Barry Taylor, and Karen Campbell. "Parental Feeding Practices Associated with Children's Eating and Weight: What Are Parents of Toddlers and Preschool Children Doing?" *Appetite* 128 (September 2018): 120–28. https://doi.org/10.1016/j.appet.2018.05.145.

Additionally, if you have a larger body . . . Mahmood, Lubna, Paloma Flores-Barrantes, Luis A. Moreno, Yannis Manios, and Esther M. Gonzalez-Gil. "The Influence of Parental

Dietary Behaviors and Practices on Children's Eating Habits." *Nutrients* 13, no. 4 (March 2021): 1138. https://doi.org/10.3390/nu13041138.

Nagging, insisting, or suggesting your child . . . Vaughn, Amber, Dianne S. Ward, Jennifer O. Fisher, Myles S. Faith, Sheryl O. Hughes, Stef Kremers, Dara R. Musher-Eizenman, Teresia M. O'Connor, Heather Patrick, and Thomas G. Power. "Fundamental Constructs in Food Parenting Practices: A Content Map to Guide Future Research." *Nutrition Reviews* 74, no. 2 (February 2016): 98–117. https://doi.org/10.1093/nutrit/nuv061.

All parents of children of varying sizes . . . Pesch, Megan H., Andrea R. Daniel, Alison L. Miller, Katherine L. Rosenblum, Danielle P. Appugliese, Julie C. Lumeng, and Niko Kaciroti. "Feeding Styles among Mothers of Low-Income Children Identified Using a Person-Centered Multi-Method Approach." *Appetite* 146 (March 2020): 104509. https://doi.org/10.1016/j.appet.2019.104509.

Overprotective feeding . . . van der Horst, Klazine, and Ester F. C. Sleddens. "Parenting Styles, Feeding Styles, and Food-Related Parenting Practices in Relation to Toddlers' Eating Styles: A Cluster-Analytic Approach." *PLOS ONE* 12, no. 5 (May 2017): e0178149. https://doi.org/10.1371/journal.pone.0178149.

Opposing the controlling feeding style . . . Vaughn, Amber, Dianne S. Ward, Jennifer O. Fisher, Myles S. Faith, Sheryl O. Hughes, Stef Kremers, Dara R. Musher-Eizenman, Teresia M. O'Connor, Heather Patrick, and Thomas G. Power. "Fundamental Constructs in Food Parenting Practices: A Content Map to Guide Future Research." *Nutrition Reviews* 74, no. 2 (Feburary 2016): 98–117. https://doi.org/10.1093/nutrit/nuv061.

As such, some children . . . Shloim, Netalie, Lisa Edelson, Nathalie Martin, and Marion M. Hetherington. "Parenting Styles, Feeding Styles, Feeding Practices, and Weight Status in 4–12 Year-Old Children: A Systematic Review of the Literature." *Frontiers in Psychology* 6 (December 2015): 1849. https://doi.org/10.3389/fpsyg.2015.01849.

A diplomatic feeding style is sensitive . . . Vaughn, Amber, Dianne S. Ward, Jennifer O. Fisher, Myles S. Faith, Sheryl O. Hughes, Stef Kremers, Dara R. Musher-Eizenman, Teresia M. O'Connor, Heather Patrick, and Thomas G. Power. "Fundamental Constructs in Food Parenting Practices: A Content Map to Guide Future Research." *Nutrition Reviews* 74, no. 2 (February 2016): 98–117. https://doi.org/10.1093/nutrit/nuv061.

Because children who are raised this way . . . Wang, Jian, Bingqian Zhu, Ruxing Wu, Yan-Shing Chang, Yang Cao, and Daqiao Zhu. "Bidirectional Associations between Parental Non-Responsive Feeding Practices and Child Eating Behaviors: A Systematic Review and Meta-Analysis of Longitudinal Prospective Studies." *Nutrients* 14, no. 9 (April 2022): 1896. https://doi.org/10.3390/nu14091896.

Or you may try to control . . . Wang, Jian, Bingqian Zhu, Ruxing Wu, Yan-Shing Chang, Yang Cao, and Daqiao Zhu. "Bidirectional Associations between Parental Non-Responsive Feeding Practices and Child Eating Behaviors: A Systematic Review and Meta-Analysis of Longitudinal Prospective Studies." *Nutrients* 14, no. 9 (April 2022): 1896. https://doi.org/10.3390/nu14091896.

Or you may try to control . . . Hudson, Paul, Pauline M. Emmett, and Caroline M. Taylor. "Pre-Pregnancy Maternal BMI Classification Is Associated with Preschool Childhood Diet Quality and Childhood Obesity in the Avon Longitudinal Study of Parents and

Children." *Public Health Nutrition* 24, no. 18 (April 2021): 6137–44. https://doi.org
/10.1017/s1368980021001476.

Or you may try to control . . . Téllez-Rojo, Martha M., Belem Trejo-Valdivia, Elizabeth
Roberts, Teresa Verenice Muñoz-Rocha, Luis F. Bautista-Arredondo, Karen E. Peterson,
and Alejandra Cantoral. "Influence of Post-Partum BMI Change on Childhood Obesity
and Energy Intake." *PLOS ONE* 14, no. 12 (December 2019): e0224830. https://doi.org
/10.1371/journal.pone.0224830.

Parents with past eating disorders . . . Martini, Maria Giulia, Manuela Barona-Martinez, and
Nadia Micali. "Eating Disorders Mothers and Their Children: A Systematic Review
of the Literature." *Archives of Women's Mental Health* 23, no. 4 (January 2020): 449–67.
https://doi.org/10.1007/s00737-020-01019-x.

Or they may not model . . . Haycraft, Emma. "Mental Health Symptoms Are Related to
Mothers' Use of Controlling and Responsive Child Feeding Practices: A Replication
and Extension Study." *Appetite* 147 (April 2020): 104523. https://doi.org/10.1016
/j.appet.2019.104523.

Food rewards are generally sweets . . . Russell, Catherine Georgina, Jillian J. Haszard, Rachael
W. Taylor, Anne-Louise M. Heath, Barry Taylor, and Karen Campbell. "Parental
Feeding Practices Associated with Children's Eating and Weight: What Are Parents
of Toddlers and Preschool Children Doing?" *Appetite* 128 (September 2018): 120–28.
https://doi.org/10.1016/j.appet.2018.05.145.

Furthermore, children may eat despite . . . Russell, Catherine Georgina, Jillian J. Haszard,
Rachael W. Taylor, Anne-Louise M. Heath, Barry Taylor, and Karen Campbell.
"Parental Feeding Practices Associated with Children's Eating and Weight: What Are
Parents of Toddlers and Preschool Children Doing?" *Appetite* 128 (September 2018):
120–28. https://doi.org/10.1016/j.appet.2018.05.145.

Making certain foods off-limits . . . Shloim, Netalie, Lisa Edelson, Nathalie Martin, and
Marion M. Hetherington. "Parenting Styles, Feeding Styles, Feeding Practices, and
Weight Status in 4–12 Year-Old Children: A Systematic Review of the Literature."
Frontiers in Psychology 6 (December 2015): 1849. https://doi.org/10.3389/fpsyg
.2015.01849.

Making food scarce . . . Ayre, S. K., Holly A. Harris, Melanie J. White, and Rebecca Byrne.
"Food-Related Parenting Practices and Styles in Households with Sibling Children:
A Scoping Review." *Appetite* 174 (July 2022): 106045. https://doi.org/10.1016/j.appet
.2022.106045.

For all children, but especially those . . . van der Horst, Klazine, and Ester F. C. Sleddens.
"Parenting Styles, Feeding Styles and Food-Related Parenting Practices in Relation to
Toddlers' Eating Styles: A Cluster-Analytic Approach." *PLOS ONE* 12, no. 5 (May 2017):
e0178149. https://doi.org/10.1371/journal.pone.0178149.

Kids who get a separate . . . Vaughn, Amber, Dianne S. Ward, Jennifer O. Fisher, Myles
S. Faith, Sheryl O. Hughes, Stef Kremers, Dara R. Musher-Eizenman, Teresia M.
O'Connor, Heather Patrick, and Thomas G. Power. "Fundamental Constructs in Food
Parenting Practices: A Content Map to Guide Future Research." *Nutrition Reviews* 74,
no. 2 (February 2016): 98–117. https://doi.org/10.1093/nutrit/nuv061.

Additionally, kids who are catered to . . . Fisher, Jennifer O., and Leann L. Birch. "Restricting Access to Palatable Foods Affects Children's Behavioral Response, Food Selection, and Intake." *The American Journal of Clinical Nutrition* 69, no. 6 (June 1999): 1264–72. https:// doi.org/10.1093/ajcn/69.6.1264.

Interestingly, parents tend to react to . . . Wolstenholme, Hazel, Colette Kelly, Marita Hennessy, and Caroline Heary. "Childhood Fussy/Picky Eating Behaviours: A Systematic Review and Synthesis of Qualitative Studies." *International Journal of Behavioral Nutrition and Physical Activity* 17, no. 1 (January 2020). https://doi.org/10.1186/s12966-019-0899-x.

Eating is your child's job . . . Ellyn Satter Institute. "Raise a Healthy Child Who Is a Joy to Feed." Accessed July 5, 2022. https://www.ellynsatterinstitute.org/how-to-feed /the-division-of-responsibility-in-feeding/.

PILLAR FIVE

Pressure to eat . . . Freitas, Ana Isabel Costa, Gabriela Albuquerque, Cláudia Silva, and Andreia Oliveira. "Appetite-Related Eating Behaviours: An Overview of Assessment Methods, Determinants and Effects on Children's Weight." *Annals of Nutrition and Metabolism* 73, no. 1 (May 2018): 19–29. https://doi.org/10.1159/000489824.

All of this is done to maintain . . . Lutter, Michael, and Eric J. Nestler. "Homeostatic and Hedonic Signals Interact in the Regulation of Food Intake." *Journal of Nutrition* 139, no. 3 (March 2009): 629–32. https://doi.org/10.3945/jn.108.097618.

Leptin helps your child . . . ScienceDirect. "Appetite Regulation." Accessed March 13, 2023. https://www.sciencedirect.com/topics/veterinary-science-and-veterinary-medicine /appetite-regulation.

Experts believe that a high amount . . . Chao, Ariana M., Ania M. Jastreboff, Marney A. White, Carlos M. Grilo, and Rajita Sinha. "Stress, Cortisol, and Other Appetite-Related Hormones: Prospective Prediction of 6-Month Changes in Food Cravings and Weight." *Obesity* 25, no. 4 (March 2017): 713–20. https://doi.org/10.1002/oby.21790.

The catch-22 is that . . . Warkentin, Sarah, Susan Carnell, and Andreia Oliveira. "Leptin at Birth and at Age 7 in Relation to Appetitive Behaviors at Age 7 and Age 10." *Hormones and Behavior* 126 (November 2020): 104842. https://doi.org/10.1016/j.yhbeh.2020.104842.

When food, especially flavors like . . . Saper, Clifford B., Tom Chou, and Joel K. Elmquist. "The Need to Feed." *Neuron* 36, no. 2 (October 2002): 199–211. https://doi.org/10.1016 /s0896-6273(02)00969-8.

When food, especially flavors like . . . Alonso-Alonso, Miguel, Stephen C. Woods, Marcia Levin Pelchat, Patricia S. Grigson, Eric Stice, I. Sadaf Farooqi, Chor San Khoo, Richard D. Mattes, and Gary K. Beauchamp. "Food Reward System: Current Perspectives and Future Research Needs." *Nutrition Reviews* 73, no. 5 (May 2015): 296–307. https://doi .org/10.1093/nutrit/nuv002.

In fact, the level of dopamine . . . Freitas, Ana Isabel Costa, Gabriela Albuquerque, Cláudia Silva, and Andreia Oliveira. "Appetite-Related Eating Behaviours: An Overview of Assessment Methods, Determinants and Effects on Children's Weight." *Annals of Nutrition and Metabolism* 73, no. 1 (May 2018): 19–29. https://doi.org/10.1159/000489824.

They may blunt fullness cues . . . Alonso-Alonso, Miguel, Stephen C. Woods, Marcia Levin Pelchat, Patricia S. Grigson, Eric Stice, I. Sadaf Farooqi, Chor San Khoo, Richard D. Mattes, and Gary K. Beauchamp. "Food Reward System: Current Perspectives and Future Research Needs." *Nutrition Reviews* 73, no. 5 (May 2015): 296–307. https://doi.org/10.1093/nutrit/nuv002.

For children to be good at regulating . . . Hayes, Jacqueline F., Dawn M. Eichen, Deanna M. Barch, and Denise E. Wilfley. "Executive Function in Childhood Obesity: Promising Intervention Strategies to Optimize Treatment Outcomes." *Appetite* 124 (May 2018): 10–23. https://doi.org/10.1016/j.appet.2017.05.040.

Children who are impulsive . . . Hayes, Jacqueline F., Dawn M. Eichen, Deanna M. Barch, and Denise E. Wilfley. "Executive Function in Childhood Obesity: Promising Intervention Strategies to Optimize Treatment Outcomes." *Appetite* 124 (May 2018): 10–23. https://doi.org/10.1016/j.appet.2017.05.040.

Preschoolers who can delay . . . Giuliani, Nicole R., and Nichole R. Kelly. "Delay of Gratification Predicts Eating in the Absence of Hunger in Preschool-Aged Children." *Frontiers in Psychology* 12 (March 2021). https://doi.org/10.3389/fpsyg.2021.650046.

Last, children who are challenged . . . Gowey, Marissa A., Crystal S. Lim, Gareth R. Dutton, Janet H. Silverstein, Marilyn Dumont-Driscoll, and David M. Janicke. "Executive Function and Dysregulated Eating Behaviors in Pediatric Obesity." *Journal of Pediatric Psychology* 43, no. 8 (September 2018): 834–45. https://doi.org/10.1093/jpepsy/jsx091.

Last, children who are challenged . . . Rhee, Kyung E., Stephanie Kessl, Michael A. Manzano, David R. Strong, and Kerri N. Boutelle. "Cluster Randomized Control Trial Promoting Child Self-Regulation around Energy-Dense Food." *Appetite* 133 (February 2019): 156–65. https://doi.org/10.1016/j.appet.2018.10.035.

This is all to say that low executive functioning . . . Gowey, Marissa A., Crystal S. Lim, Gareth R. Dutton, Janet H. Silverstein, Marilyn Dumont-Driscoll, and David M. Janicke. "Executive Function and Dysregulated Eating Behaviors in Pediatric Obesity." *Journal of Pediatric Psychology* 43, no. 8 (September 2018): 834–45. https://doi.org/10.1093/jpepsy/jsx091.

The Spectrum of Appetite Traits in Children (table) Wardle, Jane, Carol Ann Guthrie, Saskia Sanderson, and Lorna Rapoport. "Development of the Children's Eating Behaviour Questionnaire." *Journal of Child Psychology and Psychiatry* 42, no. 7 (October 2001): 963–70. https://doi.org/10.1111/1469-7610.00792.

In fact, food responsiveness . . . Llewellyn, Clare H., Cornelia H. M. van Jaarsveld, Laura Johnson, Susan Carnell, and Jane Wardle. "Nature and Nurture in Infant Appetite: Analysis of the Gemini Twin Birth Cohort." *The American Journal of Clinical Nutrition* 91, no. 5 (May 2010): 1172–79. https://doi.org/10.3945/ajcn.2009.28868.

Slowness in eating . . . Llewellyn, Clare H., Cornelia H. M. van Jaarsveld, Laura Johnson, Susan Carnell, and Jane Wardle. "Nature and Nurture in Infant Appetite: Analysis of the Gemini Twin Birth Cohort." *The American Journal of Clinical Nutrition* 91, no. 5 (May 2010): 1172–79. https://doi.org/10.3945/ajcn.2009.28868.

Variations in the appetite . . . van Jaarsveld, Cornelia H. M., Clare H. Llewellyn, Laura Johnson, and Jane Wardle. "Prospective Associations between Appetitive Traits and

Weight Gain in Infancy." *The American Journal of Clinical Nutrition* 94 (6): 1562–67. https://doi.org/10.3945/ajcn.111.015818.

One study looked at . . . van Jaarsveld, Cornelia H. M., David Boniface, Clare H. Llewellyn, and Jane Wardle. "Appetite and Growth." *JAMA Pediatrics* 168, no. 4 (April 2014): 345. https://doi.org/10.1001/jamapediatrics.2013.4951.

Furthermore, other researchers . . . Boutelle, Kerri N., Michael A. Manzano, and Dawn M. Eichen. "Appetitive Traits as Targets for Weight Loss: The Role of Food Cue Responsiveness and Satiety Responsiveness." *Physiology & Behavior* 224 (October 2020): 113018. https://doi.org/10.1016/j.physbeh.2020.113018.

There's a genetic heritability . . . Llewellyn, Clare, and Alison Fildes. "Behavioural Susceptibility Theory: Professor Jane Wardle and the Role of Appetite in Genetic Risk of Obesity." *Current Obesity Reports* 6, no. 1 (February 2017): 38–45. https://doi.org/10.1007/s13679-017-0247-x.

Children who inherit an "avid appetite," . . . Nederkoorn, Chantal, Fania C. M. Dassen, Loes Franken, Christine Resch, and Katrijn Houben. "Impulsivity and Overeating in Children in the Absence and Presence of Hunger." *Appetite* 93 (October 2015): 57–61. https://doi.org/10.1016/j.appet.2015.03.032.

Long-term activation of cortisol . . . Mayo Clinic Staff. "Chronic Stress Puts Your Health at Risk." Mayo Clinic. Last modified on August 1, 2023. https://www.mayoclinic.org/healthy-lifestyle/stress-management/in-depth/stress/art-20046037.

Chronic stress may stimulate . . . Lutter, Michael, and Eric J. Nestler. "Homeostatic and Hedonic Signals Interact in the Regulation of Food Intake." *Journal of Nutrition* 139, no. 3 (March 2009): 629–32. https://doi.org/10.3945/jn.108.097618.

Children who wake up with high . . . Michels, Nathalie, Isabelle Sioen, Caroline Braet, Inge Huybrechts, Barbara Vanaelst, Maike Wolters, and Stefaan De Henauw. "Relation between Salivary Cortisol as Stress Biomarker and Dietary Pattern in Children." *Psychoneuroendocrinology* 38, no. 9 (September 2013): 1512–20. https://doi.org/10.1016/j.psyneuen.2012.12.020.

Children who turn to food . . . Jalo, Elli, Hanna Konttinen, Henna Vepsäläinen, Jean-Philippe Chaput, Gang Hu, Carol Maher, José Maia, et al. "Emotional Eating, Health Behaviours, and Obesity in Children: A 12-Country Cross-Sectional Study." *Nutrients* 11, no. 2 (Feburary 2019): 351. https://doi.org/10.3390/nu11020351.

Of course, both why kids eat . . . Miller, Alison L., and Julie C. Lumeng. "Pathways of Association from Stress to Obesity in Early Childhood." *Obesity* 26, no. 7 (April 2018): 1117–24. https://doi.org/10.1002/oby.22155.

Studies suggest that children between the ages . . . Seymour, Karen E., Shauna P. Reinblatt, Leora Benson, and Susan Carnell. "Overlapping Neurobehavioral Circuits in ADHD, Obesity, and Binge Eating: Evidence from Neuroimaging Research." *CNS Spectrums* 20, no. 4 (June 2015): 401–11. https://doi.org/10.1017/s1092852915000383.

Especially in children who are selective . . . Galloway, Amy T., Laura M. Fiorito, Lori A. Francis, and Leann L. Birch. "'Finish Your Soup': Counterproductive Effects of Pressuring Children to Eat on Intake and Affect." *Appetite* 46, no. 3 (May 2006): 318–23. https://doi.org/10.1016/j.appet.2006.01.019.

Girls had a higher prevalence . . . López-Gil, José Francisco, Antonio García-Hermoso, Lee Smith, Joseph Firth, Mike Trott, Arthur Eumann Mesas, Estela Jiménez-López, Héctor Gutiérrez-Espinoza, Pedro J. Tárraga-López, and Desirée Victoria-Montesinos. "Global Proportion of Disordered Eating in Children and Adolescents." *JAMA Pediatrics* 177, no. 4 (February 2023): 363. https://doi.org/10.1001/jamapediatrics .2022.5848.

Boredom, particularly, is a predictor of . . . Ahlich, Erica, and Diana Rancourt. "Boredom Proneness, Interoception, and Emotional Eating." *Appetite* 178 (November 2022): 106167. https://doi.org/10.1016/j.appet.2022.106167.

EAH was reported in girls . . . Fisher, Jennifer O., and Leann L. Birch. "Restricting Access to Palatable Foods Affects Children's Behavioral Response, Food Selection, and Intake." *The American Journal of Clinical Nutrition* 69, no. 6 (June 1999): 1264–72. https://doi .org/10.1093/ajcn/69.6.1264.

Today, and for a variety of reasons . . . Schultink, Janneke M., J. H. M. de Vries, Victoire W. T. de Wild, Merel S. van Vliet, Shelley M. C. van der Veek, Vanessa E. G. Martens, C. De Graaf, and Gerry Jager. "Eating in the Absence of Hunger in 18-Month-Old Children in a Home Setting." *Pediatric Obesity* 16, no. 11 (May 2021): e12800. https:// doi.org/10.1111/ijpo.12800.

Mindful eating may improve appetite . . . Keck-Kester, Terrah, Lina Huerta-Saenz, Ryan Spotts, Laura Duda, and Nazia Raja-Khan. "Do Mindfulness Interventions Improve Obesity Rates in Children and Adolescents: A Review of the Evidence." *Diabetes, Metabolic Syndrome and Obesity: Targets and Therapy* 14 (November 2021): 4621–29. https://doi.org/10.2147/dmso.s220671.

It turns out that when kids enjoy . . . Bédard, Alexandra, Pierre-Olivier Lamarche, Lucie-Maude Grégoire, Catherine Trudel-Guy, Véronique Provencher, Sophie Desroches, and Simone Lemieux. "Can Eating Pleasure Be a Lever for Healthy Eating? A Systematic Scoping Review of Eating Pleasure and Its Links with Dietary Behaviors and Health." *PLOS ONE* 15, no. 12 (December 2020): e0244292. https://doi.org/10.1371/journal .pone.0244292.

They're also less likely to be emotional . . . Linardon, Jake, Tracy L. Tylka, and Matthew Fuller-Tyszkiewicz. "Intuitive Eating and Its Psychological Correlates: A Meta-Analysis." *International Journal of Eating Disorders* 54, no. 7 (March 2021): 1073–98. https://doi.org /10.1002/eat.23509.

However, if your child is naturally food-responsive . . . Boutelle, Kerri N., Michael A. Manzano, and Dawn M. Eichen. "Appetitive Traits as Targets for Weight Loss: The Role of Food Cue Responsiveness and Satiety Responsiveness." *Physiology & Behavior* 224 (October 2020): 113018. https://doi.org/10.1016/j.physbeh.2020.113018.

PILLAR SIX

A nutrient-rich diet is a goal . . . USDA. "Purpose of the *Dietary Guidelines*." Accessed January 24, 2022. https://www.dietaryguidelines.gov/about-dietary-guidelines /purpose-dietary-guidelines.

A snapshot of kids' eating . . . USDA. "Dietary Guidelines for Americans, 2020–2025." 164. https://www.dietaryguidelines.gov/sites/default/files/2021-03/Dietary_Guidelines_for _Americans-2020-2025.pdf.

You can find more in-depth information . . . USDA. "MyPlate." Accessed January 24, 2022. https://www.myplate.gov/.

Scientists have even found that . . . Chambers, Lucy, Keri McCrickerd, and Martin R. Yeomans. "Optimising Foods for Satiety." *Trends in Food Science and Technology* 41, no. 2 (February 2015): 149–60. https://doi.org/10.1016/j.tifs.2014.10.007.

Body temperature increases . . . Westerterp, Klaas R. "Diet Induced Thermogenesis." *Nutrition & Metabolism* 1, no. 1 (August 2004) 5. https://doi.org/10.1186/1743-7075-1-5.

A protein-rich meal . . . Arguin, Hélène, Angelo Tremblay, John Blundell, Jean-Pierre Després, Denis Richard, Benoît Lamarche, and Vicky Drapeau. "Impact of a Non-Restrictive Satiating Diet on Anthropometrics, Satiety Responsiveness and Eating Behaviour Traits in Obese Men Displaying a High or a Low Satiety Phenotype." *British Journal of Nutrition* 118, no. 9 (November 2017): 750–60. https://doi.org/10.1017 /s0007114517002549.

However, when the diet emphasizes . . . Arguin, Hélène, Angelo Tremblay, John Blundell, Jean-Pierre Després, Denis Richard, Benoît Lamarche, and Vicky Drapeau. "Impact of a Non-Restrictive Satiating Diet on Anthropometrics, Satiety Responsiveness and Eating Behaviour Traits in Obese Men Displaying a High or a Low Satiety Phenotype." *British Journal of Nutrition* 118, no. 9 (November 2017): 750–60. https://doi.org/10.1017 /s0007114517002549.

The most common nutrient deficiencies . . . USDA. "Dietary Guidelines for Americans, 2020–2025." https://www.dietaryguidelines.gov/sites/default/files/2021-03/Dietary _Guidelines_for_Americans-2020-2025.pdf.

For children with larger bodies who have a vitamin D deficiency . . . Zakharova, Irina, Leonid Klimov, Victoria Kuryaninova, Irina Nikitina, Svetlana Malyavskaya, Svetlana Dolbnya, Anna Kasyanova, et al. "Vitamin D Insufficiency in Overweight and Obese Children and Adolescents." *Frontiers in Endocrinology* 10 (March 2019). https://doi.org/10.3389 /fendo.2019.00103.

Additionally, studies show the omega-3 index . . . Wu, Shaojing, Chunhong Zhu, Zhen Wang, Shumei Wang, Peng Yuan, Tao Song, Xiaoming Hou, and Zhixian Lei. "Effects of Fish Oil Supplementation on Cardiometabolic Risk Factors in Overweight or Obese Children and Adolescents: A Meta-Analysis of Randomized Controlled Trials." *Frontiers in Pediatrics* 9 (April 2021). https://doi.org/10.3389/fped.2021.604469.

This is a common scenario in selective eaters . . . Wolstenholme, Hazel, Colette Kelly, Marita Hennessy, and Caroline Heary. "Childhood Fussy/Picky Eating Behaviours: A Systematic Review and Synthesis of Qualitative Studies." *International Journal of Behavioral Nutrition and Physical Activity* 17, no. 1 (January 2020). https://doi.org/10.1186/s12966-019-0899-x.

Iron deficiency and anemia experienced in infancy . . . Cusick, Sarah E., Michael Georgieff, and Raghavendra Rao. "Approaches for Reducing the Risk of Early-Life Iron

Deficiency-Induced Brain Dysfunction in Children." *Nutrients* 10, no. 2 (February 2018): 227. https://doi.org/10.3390/nu10020227.

Furthermore, 20 percent of the children . . . No Kid Hungry. "How Many Kids in the United States Live with Hunger?" Accessed October 25, 2023. https://www.nokidhungry .org/blog/how-many-kids-united-states-live-hunger.

Surprisingly, even financially stable households . . . Tufts. "Ultraprocessed Foods Now Comprise 2/3 of Calories in Children and Teen Diets." *Tufts Now.* Published August 10, 2021; accessed January 25, 2022. https://now.tufts.edu/news-releases/ultraprocessed-foods -now-comprise-23-calories-children-and-teen-diets.

For any child with good health . . . Koliaki, Chrysi, Theodoros Spinos, Marianna Spinou, Maria-Eugenia Brinia, Dimitra Mitsopoulou, and Nicholas Katsilambros. "Defining the Optimal Dietary Approach for Safe, Effective and Sustainable Weight Loss in Overweight and Obese Adults." *Healthcare* 6, no. 3 (June 2018): 73. https://doi.org /10.3390/healthcare6030073.

Scientists believe mood affects our food . . . AlAmmar, Welayah A., Fatima H. Albeesh, and Rabie Khattab. "Food and Mood: the Correspondent Effect." *Current Nutrition Reports* 9, no. 3 (July 2020): 296–308. https://doi.org/10.1007/s13668-020-00331-3.

For instance, complex carbohydrates . . . Shabbir, Faisal, Akash Patel, Charles Mattison, Saswata Bose, Raathathulaksi Krishnamohan, Emily A. Sweeney, Sarina Sandhu, et al. "Effect of Diet on Serotonergic Neurotransmission in Depression." *Neurochemistry International* 62, no. 3 (February 2013): 324–29. https://doi.org/10.1016/j.neuint.2012.12.014.

Even fruits and vegetables . . . Mujcic, Redzo, and Andrew J. Oswald. "Evolution of Well-Being and Happiness after Increases in Consumption of Fruit and Vegetables." *American Journal of Public Health* 106, no. 8 (August 2016): 1504–10. Published October 28, 2019. https://doi.org/10.2105/ajph.2016.303260.

Nutrition research has also identified . . . HealthyChildren.org. "American Academy of Pediatrics Looks at Use of Nonnutritive Sweeteners by Children." Accessed March 2, 2022. https://www.healthychildren.org/English/news/Pages/The-Use-of-Nonnutritive -Sweeteners-in-Children.aspx.

Nutrition research has also identified . . . LaChance, Laura, and Drew Ramsey. "Antidepressant Foods: An Evidence-Based Nutrient Profiling System for Depression." *World Journal of Psychiatry* 8, no. 3 (September 2018): 97–104. https://doi.org/10.5498/wjp.v8.i3.97.

Synbiotics are combinations of . . . Pandey, Kavita, S. R. Naik, and Babu V. Vakil. "Probiotics, Prebiotics and Synbiotics—A Review." *Journal of Food Science and Technology* 52, no. 12 (July 2015): 7577–87. https://doi.org/10.1007/s13197-015-1921-1.

In children ages five to seven, the DASH diet . . . Zafarmand, Mohammad Hadi, Marit Spanjer, Mary Nicolaou, Hanneke A. H. Wijnhoven, Barbera D. C. Van Schaik, André G. Uitterlinden, Harold Snieder, and Tanja G. M. Vrijkotte. "Influence of Dietary Approaches to Stop Hypertension-Type Diet, Known Genetic Variants and Their Interplay on Blood Pressure in Early Childhood." *Hypertension* 75, no. 1 (January 2020): 59–70. https://doi.org/10.1161/hypertensionaha.118.12292.

The National Heart, Lung, and Blood Institute also offers . . . NHLBI. "What Is High Blood Pressure?" NIH: National Heart, Lung, and Blood Institute. Last modified on March 24, 2022. https://www.nhlbi.nih.gov/health-topics/high-blood-pressure.

The Mediterranean diet has been identified . . . D'Innocenzo, Santa, Carlotta Biagi, and Marcello Lanari. "Obesity and the Mediterranean Diet: A Review of Evidence of the Role and Sustainability of the Mediterranean Diet." *Nutrients* 11, no. 6 (June 2019): 1306. https://doi.org/10.3390/nu11061306.

The Mediterranean diet has been identified . . . Notario-Barandiaran, Leyre, Desirée Valera-Gran, Sandra González-Palacios, Manuela García-De-La-Hera, Sílvia Fernández-Barrés, Eva Pereda Pereda, Ana Fernández-Somoano, et al. "High Adherence to a Mediterranean Diet at Age 4 Reduces Overweight, Obesity and Abdominal Obesity Incidence in Children at the Age of 8." *International Journal of Obesity* 44, no. 9 (March 2020): 1906–17. https://doi.org/10.1038/s41366-020-0557-z.

Results in a diet lower . . . Motevalli, Mohamad, Clemens Drenowatz, Derrick Tanous, Naim Akhtar Khan, and Katharina Wirnitzer. "Management of Childhood Obesity— Time to Shift from Generalized to Personalized Intervention Strategies." *Nutrients* 13, no. 4 (April 2021): 1200. https://doi.org/10.3390/nu13041200.

Experts argue about which foods . . . Braesco, Véronique, Isabelle Souchon, Patrick Sauvant, Typhaine Haurogné, Matthieu Maillot, Catherine Féart, and Nicole Darmon. "Ultra-Processed Foods: How Functional Is the NOVA System?" *European Journal of Clinical Nutrition* 76, no. 9 (March 2022): 1245–53. https://doi.org/10.1038/s41430-022-01099-1.

They cap sugar at five to ten teaspoons a day . . . Austrian Agency for Health and Food Safety. "WHO Sugar Recommendations" *AGES.* Last modified October 10, 2023. https://www.ages.at/en/human/nutrition-food/nutrition-recommendations/who-sugar-recommendations#:~:text=WHO%20sugar%20recommendations%3A%20max.,at%20all%20stages%20of%20life.

The 2020 Dietary Guidelines for Americans agree, suggesting . . . USDA. "Dietary Guidelines for Americans, 2020–2025." Accessed December 1, 2022. https://www.dietaryguidelines.gov/sites/default/files/2021-03/Dietary_Guidelines_for_Americans-2020-2025.pdf.

Toddlers and preschoolers are consuming . . . CDC. "Know Your Limit for Added Sugars." Accessed November 28, 2021. https://www.cdc.gov/nutrition/data-statistics/added-sugars.html.

Long-term studies show kids develop . . . Baker-Smith, Carissa, Sarah D. de Ferranti, William J. Cochran, Committee on Nutrition, Section on Gastroenterology, Hepatology, and Nutrition. "The Use of Nonnutritive Sweeteners in Children." *Pediatrics* 144, no. 5 (November 2019): e20192765. https://doi.org/10.1542/peds.2019-2765.

While children are consuming fewer sodas . . . Dai, Jane, Mark J. Soto, Caroline Dunn, and Sara N. Bleich. "Trends and Patterns in Sugar-Sweetened Beverage Consumption among Children and Adults by Race and/or Ethnicity, 2003–2018." *Public Health Nutrition* 24, no. 9 (April 2021): 2405–10. https://doi.org/10.1017/s1368980021001580.

But eating larger portions doesn't necessarily . . . Hetherington, Marion M., Pam Blundell-Birtill, Samantha J. Caton, Joanne E. Cecil, Charlotte Evans, Barbara J. Rolls, and Tang Tang. "Understanding the Science of Portion Control and the Art of Downsizing."

Proceedings of the Nutrition Society 77, no. 3 (May 2018): 347–55. https://doi.org/10.1017 /s0029665118000435.

In fact, a review study looked at cooking . . . DeCosta, Patricia, Per Møller, Michael Frøst, and Annemarie Olsen. "Changing Children's Eating Behaviour—A Review of Experimental Research." *Appetite* 113 (June 2017): 327–57. https://doi.org/10.1016 /j.appet.2017.03.004.

Studies of school gardens . . . DeCosta, Patricia, Per Møller, Michael Frøst, and Annemarie Olsen. "Changing Children's Eating Behaviour—A Review of Experimental Research." *Appetite* 113 (June 2017): 327–57. https://doi.org/10.1016/j.appet.2017.03.004.

Studies are ambivalent about food tastings . . . DeCosta, Patricia, Per Møller, Michael Frøst, and Annemarie Olsen. "Changing Children's Eating Behaviour—A Review of Experimental Research." *Appetite* 113 (June 2017): 327–57. https://doi.org/10.1016 /j.appet.2017.03.004.

PILLAR SEVEN

In toddlers and preschoolers, time in front of screens . . . Common Sense. "The Common Sense Census: Media Use by Kids Age Zero to Eight, 2020." Accessed November 23, 2020. https://www.commonsensemedia.org/research/the-common-sense-census-media -use-by-kids-age-zero-to-eight-2020.

Eight- to twelve-year-old children . . . Cardoso-Leite, Pedro, Albert Buchard, Isabel Tissieres, Dominic Mussack, and Daphne Bavelier. "Media Use, Attention, Mental Health and Academic Performance among 8 to 12 Year Old Children." *PLOS ONE* 16, no. 11 (November 2021): e0259163. https://doi.org/10.1371/journal.pone.0259163.

Shockingly, media exposure . . . Chassiakos, Yolanda Reid, Jenny Radesky, Dimitri A. Christakis, Megan A. Moreno, Corinn Cross, David L. Hill, Nusheen Ameenuddin, et al. "Children and Adolescents and Digital Media." *Pediatrics* 138, no. 5 (November 2016): e20162593. https://doi.org/10.1542/peds.2016-2593.

Unfortunately, these outlets may lack educational . . . Common Sense. "The Common Sense Census: Media Use by Tweens and Teens, 2021." Published March 9, 2022; accessed January 20, 2023. https://www.commonsensemedia.org/research/the-common-sense -census-media-use-by-tweens-and-teens-2021.

Nearly across the board, engagement with screens . . . McClain, Colleen. "How Parents' Views of Their Kids' Screen Time, Social Media Use Changed during COVID-19." Pew Research Center: Children & Tech. April 28, 2022. https://www.pewresearch.org /fact-tank/2022/04/28/how-parents-views-of-their-kids-screen-time-social-media-use -changed-during-covid-19/.

Another recent survey measured screen time . . . Kroshus, Emily, Pooja Tandon, Chuan Zhou, Alice Johnson, Mary Kathleen Steiner, and Dimitri A. Christakis. "Problematic Child Media Use during the COVID-19 Pandemic." *Pediatrics* 150, no. 3 (August 2022): e2021055190. https://doi.org/10.1542/peds.2021-055190.

YouTube leads the pack in popularity . . . Atske, Sara. "Teens, Social Media and Technology 2022." Pew Research Center: Internet, Science & Tech. Last modified April 28, 2022.

https://www.pewresearch.org/internet/2022/08/10/teens-social-media-and-technology-2022/.

Studies show that passive learning . . . Ehmke, Rachel, and Donna Wick. "Media Guidelines for Kids of All Ages." *Child Mind Institute.* Last modified on November 20, 2023. https://childmind.org/article/media-guidelines-for-kids-of-all-ages/.

School-age children who engage more with media . . . Cardoso-Leite, Pedro, Albert Buchard, Isabel Tissieres, Dominic Mussack, and Daphne Bavelier. "Media Use, Attention, Mental Health and Academic Performance among 8 to 12 Year Old Children." *PLOS ONE* 16, no. 11 (November 2021): e0259163. https://doi.org/10.1371/journal.pone.0259163.

The more hours of video game play . . . Cardoso-Leite, Pedro, Albert Buchard, Isabel Tissieres, Dominic Mussack, and Daphne Bavelier. "Media Use, Attention, Mental Health and Academic Performance among 8 to 12 Year Old Children." *PLOS ONE* 16, no. 11 (November 2021): e0259163. https://doi.org/10.1371/journal.pone.0259163.

But gaming may be beneficial . . . Kovess-Masfety, Viviane, Katherine M. Keyes, Ava Hamilton, Gregory D. Hanson, Adina Bitfoi, Dietmar Gölitz, Ceren Koç, et al. "Is Time Spent Playing Video Games Associated with Mental Health, Cognitive and Social Skills in Young Children?" *Social Psychiatry and Psychiatric Epidemiology* 51, no. 3 (February 2016): 349–57. https://doi.org/10.1007/s00127-016-1179-6.

When toddlers and preschoolers view media . . . Oflu, Ayşe Tolunay, Özlem Tezol, Seda Yalcin, Deniz Yildiz, Nilgün Çaylan, Dilşad Foto Özdemir, Şeyma Çiçek, and Meryem Erat Nergiz. "Excessive Screen Time Is Associated with Emotional Lability in Preschool Children." *Archivos Argentinos de Pediatría* 119, no. 2 (September 2021): 106–13. https://doi.org/10.5546/aap.2021.eng.106.

And in the preteen years, high media engagement . . . Oswald, Tassia K., Alice Rumbold, Sophie G. E. Kedzior, and Vivienne Moore. "Psychological Impacts of 'Screen Time' and 'Green Time' for Children and Adolescents: A Systematic Scoping Review." *PLOS ONE* 15, no. 9 (September 2020): e0237725. https://doi.org/10.1371/journal.pone.0237725.

Furthermore, watching videos is linked to . . . Fors, Payton, and Deanna M. Barch. "Differential Relationships of Child Anxiety and Depression to Child Report and Parent Report of Electronic Media Use." *Child Psychiatry & Human Development* 50, no. 6 (May 2019): 907–17. https://doi.org/10.1007/s10578-019-00892-7.

It's a way to ease these negative sensations . . . Epkins, Catherine C. "Experiential Avoidance and Anxiety Sensitivity: Independent and Specific Associations with Children's Depression, Anxiety, and Social Anxiety Symptoms." *Journal of Psychopathology and Behavioral Assessment* 38. no. 1 (July 2015): 124–35. https://doi.org/10.1007/s10862-015-9502-1.

Ironically, engaging with social media . . . Fors, Payton, and Deanna M. Barch. "Differential Relationships of Child Anxiety and Depression to Child Report and Parent Report of Electronic Media Use." *Child Psychiatry & Human Development* 50, no. 6 (May 2019): 907–17. https://doi.org/10.1007/s10578-019-00892-7.

Being outside in nature . . . Oswald, Tassia K., Alice Rumbold, Sophie G. E. Kedzior, and Vivienne Moore. "Psychological Impacts of 'Screen Time' and 'Green Time' for Children and Adolescents: A Systematic Scoping Review." *PLOS ONE* 15, no. 9 (September 2020): e0237725. https://doi.org/10.1371/journal.pone.0237725.

Unfortunately, US kids spend fewer . . . DJ Case and Associates "The Nature of Americans National Report: Disconnection and Recommendations for Reconnection." Accessed November 21, 2022. https://natureofamericans.org/findings/viz/media-use-increases -while-outdoor-time-decreases-among-older-children.

In four- to eighteen-year-olds, watching television . . . Adelantado-Renau, Mireia, Diego Moliner-Urdiales, Iván Cavero-Redondo, Maria Reyes Beltran-Valls, Vicente Martínez-Vizcaíno, and Celia Álvarez-Bueno. "Association between Screen Media Use and Academic Performance among Children and Adolescents." *JAMA Pediatrics* 173, no. 11 (September 2019): 1058. https://doi.org/10.1001/jamapediatrics.2019.3176.

And it's almost a guarantee . . . Martin, Katie, Jana Bednarz, and Edoardo Aromataris. "Interventions to Control Children's Screen Use and Their Effect on Sleep: A Systematic Review and Meta-Analysis." *Journal of Sleep Research* 30, no. 3 (June 2020): e13130. https://doi.org/10.1111/jsr.13130.

Efforts at reducing screen time . . . Zhang, Ping, Xian Tang, Xin Peng, Guang Hao, Sheng-Wei Luo, and Xiaohua Liang. "Effect of Screen Time Intervention on Obesity among Children and Adolescent: A Meta-Analysis of Randomized Controlled Studies." *Preventive Medicine* 157 (April 2022): 107014. https://doi.org/10.1016/j.ypmed.2022 .107014.

Screen Time Recommendations for Children (table) HealthyChildren.org. "Where We Stand: Screen Time." Last modified December 13, 2023. https://www.healthychildren.org /English/family-life/Media/Pages/Where-We-Stand-TV-Viewing-Time.aspx.

According to a recent survey . . . Nadeem, Reem. "Parenting Kids in the Age of Screens, Social Media and Digital Devices." Pew Research Center: Internet, Science & Tech. Published July 28, 2020; accessed November 30, 2022. https://www.pewresearch.org /internet/2020/07/28/parenting-children-in-the-age-of-screens/.

Parents with high screen use . . . Tang, Lisa, Gerarda Darlington, David W. L. Ma, and Jess Haines. "Mothers' and Fathers' Media Parenting Practices Associated with Young Children's Screen-Time: A Cross-Sectional Study." *BMC Obesity* 5, no. 1 (December 2018). https://doi.org/10.1186/s40608-018-0214-4.

Parental self-efficacy is key . . . Kieslinger, Katrin, Olivia Wartha, Olga Pollatos, Jürgen M. Steinacker, and Susanne Kobel. "Parental Self-Efficacy—A Predictor of Children's Health Behaviors? Its Impact on Children's Physical Activity and Screen Media Use and Potential Interaction Effect within a Health Promotion Program." *Frontiers in Psychology* 12 (August 2021). https://doi.org/10.3389/fpsyg.2021.712796.

Parents who have confidence . . . Kieslinger, Katrin, Olivia Wartha, Olga Pollatos, Jürgen M. Steinacker, and Susanne Kobel. "Parental Self-Efficacy—A Predictor of Children's Health Behaviors? Its Impact on Children's Physical Activity and Screen Media Use and Potential Interaction Effect within a Health Promotion Program." *Frontiers in Psychology* 12 (August 2021). https://doi.org/10.3389/fpsyg.2021.712796.

More than half of parents . . . Nadeem, Reem. "Parenting Kids in the Age of Screens, Social Media and Digital Devices." Pew Research Center: Internet, Science & Tech. Published July 28, 2020; accessed November 30, 2022. https://www.pewresearch.org /internet/2020/07/28/parenting-children-in-the-age-of-screens/.

One study found that chaotic households . . . Emond, Jennifer A., Lucy K. Tantum, Diane Gilbert-Diamond, Sunny Jung Kim, Reina K. Lansigan, and Sara Benjamin Neelon. "Household Chaos and Screen Media Use among Preschool-Aged Children: A Cross-Sectional Study." *BMC Public Health* 18, no. 1 (October 2018). https://doi.org/10.1186/s12889-018-6113-2.

The incidence of eating disorders . . . Devoe, Dan, Angela Han, Alida Anderson, Debra K. Katzman, Scott B. Patten, Andrea Soumbasis, Jordyn Flanagan, et al. "The Impact of the COVID-19 Pandemic on Eating Disorders: A Systematic Review." *International Journal of Eating Disorders* 56, no. 1 (April 2022): 5–25. https://doi.org/10.1002/eat.23704.

And it keeps feeding . . . Hobbs, Tawnell D., Rob Barry, and Yoree Koh. "'The Corpse Bride Diet': How TikTok Inundates Teens with Eating-Disorder Videos." *The Wall Street Journal.* Accessed December 19, 2021. https://www.wsj.com/articles/how-tiktok-inundates-teens-with-eating-disorder-videos-11639754848.

Furthermore, in 2021, Facebook, TikTok, and Instagram . . . Allyn, Bobby. "4 Takeaways from the Senate Child Safety Hearing with YouTube, Snapchat and TikTok." *NPR.* Accessed March 14, 2023. https://www.npr.org/2021/10/26/1049267501/snapchat-tiktok-youtube-congress-child-safety-hearing.

Kids as young as eight years . . . Common Sense. "The Common Sense Census: Media Use by Kids Age Zero to Eight, 2020." Accessed November 23, 2022. https://www.commonsensemedia.org/research/the-common-sense-census-media-use-by-kids-age-zero-to-eight-2020.

Some companies have been called out . . . "5Rights Foundation." Accessed February 17, 2023. https://5rightsfoundation.com/.

Both boys and girls are affected . . . De Coen, Jolien, Sandra Verbeken, and Lien Goossens. "Media Influence Components as Predictors of Children's Body Image and Eating Problems: A Longitudinal Study of Boys and Girls during Middle Childhood." *Body Image* 37 (June 2021): 204–13. https://doi.org/10.1016/j.bodyim.2021.03.001.

Twenty-three percent of middle and high schoolers . . . Hamm, Michele P., Amanda S. Newton, Annabritt Chisholm, Jocelyn Shulhan, Andrea Milne, Purnima Sundar, Heather Ennis, Shannon D. Scott, and Lisa Hartling. "Prevalence and Effect of Cyberbullying on Children and Young People." *JAMA Pediatrics* 169, no. 8 (August 2015): 770. https://doi.org/10.1001/jamapediatrics.2015.0944.

Victims of cyberbullying . . . John, Ann, Alexander Charles Glendenning, Amanda Marchant, Paul Montgomery, Anne Stewart, Sophie Wood, Kenneth E. Lloyd, and Keith Hawton. "Self-Harm, Suicidal Behaviours, and Cyberbullying in Children and Young People: Systematic Review." *Journal of Medical Internet Research* 20, no. 4 (April 2018): e129. https://doi.org/10.2196/jmir.9044.

Children with larger bodies are targets . . . Waasdorp, Tracy Evian, Krista R. Mehari, and Catherine P. Bradshaw. "Obese and Overweight Youth: Risk for Experiencing Bullying Victimization and Internalizing Symptoms." *American Journal of Orthopsychiatry* 88, no. 4 (January 2018): 483–91. https://doi.org/10.1037/ort0000294.

Furthermore, boys, rather than girls . . . Fowler, Lauren A., Chelsea L. Kracht, Kara D. Denstel, and Tiffany M. Stewart. "Bullying Experiences, Body Esteem, Body Dissatisfaction, and the Moderating Role of Weight Status among Adolescents." *Journal of Adolescence* 91, no. 1 (July 2021): 59–70. https://doi.org/10.1016/j.adolescence.2021.07.006.

Kids with larger bodies tend to deal with . . . Walsh, Órla, Elizabeth Dettmer, Andrea Regina, Linlei Ye, Jennifer Christian, Jill Hamilton, and Alene Toulany. "'I Don't Want Them to Think that What They Said Matters': How Treatment-Seeking Adolescents with Severe Obesity Cope with Weight-Based Victimization." *Clinical Obesity* 11, no. 3 (January 2021): e12437. https://doi.org/10.1111/cob.12437.

Television is the main source of marketing . . . UConn Rudd Center for Food Policy and Health. "Food Marketing." Accessed November 30, 2022. https://uconnruddcenter.org /research/food-marketing/.

Although there's been a major downshift . . . UConn Rudd Center for Food Policy and Health. "Food Marketing." Accessed November 30, 2022. https://uconnruddcenter.org/research /food-marketing/.

The American Academy of Pediatrics (AAP) advises parents . . . Korioth, Trista. "Family Media Plan Helps Parents Set Boundaries for Kids." *AAP News.* October 21, 2016. https://publications.aap.org/aapnews/news/9082/Family-Media-Plan-helps-parents-set -boundaries-for.

Mike Caulfield, a digital literacy expert . . . Caulfield, Mike. "SIFT (The Four Moves)." *Hapgood.* Accessed December 9, 2022. https://hapgood.us/2019/06/19/sift-the-four -moves/.

You'll also find them available on . . . Habas, Cathy. "2023 Best Parental Control Apps & Software." *SafeWise.* Last modified September 7, 2023. https://www.safewise.com /resources/parental-control-filters-buyers-guide/.

Even health-promoting media campaigns . . . Puhl, Rebecca M., and Leah M. Lessard. "Weight Stigma in Youth: Prevalence, Consequences, and Considerations for Clinical Practice." *Current Obesity Reports* 9, no. 4 (October 2020): 402–11. https://doi.org /10.1007/s13679-020-00408-8.

PILLAR EIGHT

This self-positivity bias contributes to . . . Asghar, Andleeb. "The Science of Self-Love: The Evidence-Based Benefits of Loving Yourself." Ness Labs. Accessed December 11, 2022. https://nesslabs.com/self-love.

Researchers have found that about . . . Bleidorn, Wiebke, Anke Hufer, Christian Kandler, Christopher J. Hopwood, and Rainer Riemann. "A Nuclear Twin Family Study of Self-Esteem." *European Journal of Personality* 32, no. 3 (May 2018): 221–32. https:// doi.org/10.1002/per.2136.

Generation Z, people born . . . The Body Shop. "Self Love Index." Accessed December 13, 2022. https://www.thebodyshop.com/en-us/about-us/activism/self-love/self-love-index /a/a00043.

Lower self-esteem may even lead . . . Orth, Ulrich. "The Lifespan Development of Self-Esteem." In *Personality Development across the Lifespan*, edited by Julie Specht, 181–95. Cambridge, MA: Academic Press, 2017. https://doi.org/10.1016/b978-0-12-804674 -6.00012-0.

Gender, school performance . . . Orth, Ulrich. "The Lifespan Development of Self-Esteem." In *Personality Development across the Lifespan*, edited by Julie Specht, 181–95. Cambridge, MA: Academic Press, 2017. https://doi.org/10.1016/b978-0-12-804674-6.00012-0.

Self-care has several benefits . . . Luis, Elkin O., Elena Bermejo-Martins, Martín Martínez, Ainize Sarrionandia, C. Cortés, Edwin Yair Oliveros, María Sol Garcés, José Victor Oron, and Pablo Fernández-Berrocal. "Relationship between Self-Care Activities, Stress and Well-Being during COVID-19 Lockdown: A Cross-Cultural Mediation Model." *BMJ Open* 11, no. 12 (December 2021): e048469. https://doi.org/10.1136/bmjopen-2020-048469.

A 2021 study found that adults who perceived more stress . . . Luis, Elkin O., Elena Bermejo-Martins, Martín Martínez, Ainize Sarrionandia, C. Cortés, Edwin Yair Oliveros, María Sol Garcés, José Victor Oron, and Pablo Fernández-Berrocal. "Relationship between Self-Care Activities, Stress and Well-Being during COVID-19 Lockdown: A Cross-Cultural Mediation Model." *BMJ Open* 11, no. 12 (December 2021): e048469. https:// doi.org/10.1136/bmjopen-2020-048469.

In a study of medical students . . . Saunders, Pamela, Rochelle E. Tractenberg, Ranjana Chaterji, Hakima Amri, Nancy Harazduk, James S. Gordon, Michael D. Lumpkin, and Aviad Haramati. "Promoting Self-Awareness and Reflection through an Experiential Mind-Body Skills Course for First Year Medical Students." *Medical Teacher* 29, no. 8 (January 2007): 778–84. https://doi.org/10.1080/01421590701509647.

In a study of medical students . . . James, Colin. "Law Student Wellbeing: Benefits of Promoting Psychological Literacy and Self-Awareness Using Mindfulness, Strengths Theory and Emotional Intelligence." *Legal Education Review* 21, no. 2 (September 2011): 217–233. https://www.academia.edu/8275714/Law_Student_Wellbeing_Benefits_of_ Promoting_Psychological_Literacy_and_Self_Awareness_Using_Mindfulness_Strengths _Theory_and_Emotional_Intelligence.

When kids disconnect from their bodies . . . Sturgess, Clea, and Danu Anthony Stinson. "Fat Embodiment for Resistance and Healing from Weight Stigma." *Body Image* 41 (June 2022): 52–57. https://doi.org/10.1016/j.bodyim.2022.02.007.

This can lead to self-loathing . . . Pearl, Raymond, and Rebecca M. Puhl. "Weight Bias Internalization and Health: A Systematic Review." *Obesity Reviews* 19, no. 8 (May 2018): 1141–63. https://doi.org/10.1111/obr.12701.

In other words, size stigma . . . Williams, Oli, and Ellen Annandale. "Weight Bias Internalization as an Embodied Process: Understanding How Obesity Stigma Gets under the Skin." *Frontiers in Psychology* 10 (April 2019). https://doi.org/10.3389 /fpsyg.2019.00953.

Shockingly, simply perceiving . . . Tomiyama, A. Janet, Deborah Carr, Ellen M. Granberg, Brenda Major, Eric Robinson, Angelina R. Sutin, and Alexandra Brewis. "How and Why Weight Stigma Drives the Obesity 'Epidemic' and Harms Health." *BMC Medicine* 16, no. 1 (August 2018). https://doi.org/10.1186/s12916-018-1116-5.

From age eight years on . . . Hendriks, Eline, Peter Muris, and Cor Meesters. "The Influence of Negative Feedback and Social Rank on Feelings of Shame and Guilt: A Vignette Study in 8- to 13-Year-Old Non-Clinical Children." *Child Psychiatry & Human Development* 53, no. 3 (February 2021): 458–68. https://doi.org/10.1007/s10578-021-01143-4.

Negative feedback of any kind . . . Bidjerano, Temi. "Self-Conscious Emotions in Response to Perceived Failure: A Structural Equation Model." *Journal of Experimental Education* 78, no. 3 (August 2010): 318–42. https://doi.org/10.1080/00220970903548079.

Negative feedback of any kind . . . Belschak, Frank D., and Deanne N. Den Hartog. "Consequences of Positive and Negative Feedback: The Impact on Emotions and Extra-Role Behaviors." *Applied Psychology* 58, no. 2 (April 2009): 274–303. https://doi.org/10.1111/j.1464-0597.2008.00336.x.

Negative feedback of any kind . . . Fourie, Melike M., Kevin G. F. Thomas, David M. Amodio, Christopher Warton, and Ernesta M. Meintjes. "Neural Correlates of Experienced Moral Emotion: An FMRI Investigation of Emotion in Response to Prejudice Feedback." *Social Neuroscience* 9, no. 2 (January 2014): 203–18. https://doi.org/10.1080/17470919.2013.878750.

Negative feedback of any kind . . . Johnson, Genevieve Marie, and Shane Connelly. "Negative Emotions in Informal Feedback: The Benefits of Disappointment and Drawbacks of Anger." *Human Relations* 67, no. 10 (June 2014): 1265–90. https://doi.org/10.1177/0018726714532856.

Kids who perceive themselves as disliked . . . Irons, Chris, and Paul Gilbert. "Evolved Mechanisms in Adolescent Anxiety and Depression Symptoms: The Role of the Attachment and Social Rank Systems." *Journal of Adolescence* 28, no. 3 (October 2004): 325–41. https://doi.org/10.1016/j.adolescence.2004.07.004.

Girls seem to be more susceptible . . . Hendriks, Eline, Peter Muris, and Cor Meesters. "The Influence of Negative Feedback and Social Rank on Feelings of Shame and Guilt: A Vignette Study in 8- to 13-Year-Old Non-Clinical Children." *Child Psychiatry & Human Development* 53, no. 3 (February 2021): 458–68. https://doi.org/10.1007/s10578-021-01143-4.

THRIVING AT EVERY SIZE, INSIDE AND OUT

Two-thirds of adults who are larger . . . Puhl, Rebecca M., Leah M. Lessard, Mary S. Himmelstein, and Gary D. Foster. "The Roles of Experienced and Internalized Weight Stigma in Healthcare Experiences: Perspectives of Adults Engaged in Weight Management across Six Countries." *PLOS ONE* 16, no. 6 (June 2021): e0251566. https://doi.org/10.1371/journal.pone.0251566.

The weight-inclusive approach *mitigates* . . . Tylka, Tracy L., Rachel A. Annunziato, Deb Burgard, Sigrún Daníelsdóttir, Ellen Shuman, Chad Davis, and Rachel M. Calogero. "The Weight-Inclusive versus Weight-Normative Approach to Health: Evaluating the Evidence for Prioritizing Well-Being over Weight Loss." *Journal of Obesity* 2014 (January 2014): 1–18. https://doi.org/10.1155/2014/983495.

Called intensive health behavior and lifestyle treatment . . . Hampl, Sarah, Sandra G. Hassink, Asheley Cockrell Skinner, Sarah Armstrong, Sarah E. Barlow, Christopher Bolling, Kimberly C. Avila Edwards, et al. "Clinical Practice Guideline for the Evaluation and Treatment of Children and Adolescents with Obesity." *Pediatrics* 151, no. 2 (January 2023). https://doi.org/10.1542/peds.2022-060640.

IHBLT is most successful when . . . Hampl, Sarah, Sandra G. Hassink, Asheley Cockrell Skinner, Sarah Armstrong, Sarah E. Barlow, Christopher Bolling, Kimberly C. Avila Edwards, et al. "Clinical Practice Guideline for the Evaluation and Treatment of Children and Adolescents with Obesity." *Pediatrics* 151, no. 2 (January 2023). https://doi.org/10.1542/peds.2022-060640.

As you've learned, changing a child's size . . . Tylka, Tracy L., Rachel A. Annunziato, Deb Burgard, Sigrún Daníelsdóttir, Ellen Shuman, Chad Davis, and Rachel M. Calogero. "The Weight-Inclusive versus Weight-Normative Approach to Health: Evaluating the Evidence for Prioritizing Well-Being over Weight Loss." *Journal of Obesity* 2014 (January 2014): 1–18. https://doi.org/10.1155/2014/983495.

Children with special health-care needs . . . Bandini, Linda G., Melissa L. Danielson, Layla Esposito, John T. Foley, Michael H. Fox, Georgia C. Frey, Richard K. Fleming, et al. "Obesity in Children with Developmental and/or Physical Disabilities." *Disability and Health Journal* 8, no. 3 (July 2015): 309–16. https://doi.org/10.1016/j.dhjo.2015.04.005.

Changes in what, when, and how much your child eats . . . Devoe, Daniel J., Angela Han, Alida Anderson, Debra K. Katzman, Scott B. Patten, Andrea Soumbasis, Jordyn Flanagan, et al. "The Impact of the COVID-19 Pandemic on Eating Disorders: A Systematic Review." *International Journal of Eating Disorders* 56, no. 1 (April 2022): 5–25. https://doi.org/10.1002/eat.23704.

In the child who hasn't rolled through . . . Patel, Meera, Sharon M. Donovan, and Soo Yeun Lee. "Considering Nature and Nurture in the Etiology and Prevention of Picky Eating: A Narrative Review." *Nutrients* 12, no. 11 (November 2020): 3409. https://doi.org/10.3390/nu12113409.

Picky eating is highly heritable . . . Cooke, Lucy, Claire M. A. Haworth, and Jane Wardle. "Genetic and Environmental Influences on Children's Food Neophobia." *The American Journal of Clinical Nutrition* 86, no. 2 (August 2007): 428–33. https://doi.org/10.1093/ajcn/86.2.428.

In children with ARFID . . . NEDA. "Statistics & Research on Eating Disorders." National Eating Disorders Association. Accessed on February 19, 2018. https://www.nationaleatingdisorders.org/statistics-research-eating-disorders.

Eating disorders have a genetic basis . . . Rienecke, Renee D. "Family-Based Treatment of Eating Disorders in Adolescents: Current Insights." *Adolescent Health, Medicine and Therapeutics* 8 (June 2017): 69–79. https://doi.org/10.2147/ahmt.s115775.

Ironically, parents often miss the signs . . . Coelho, Jennifer S., Janet Suen, Sheila K. Marshall, Alex Burns, Pei-Yoong Lam, and Josie Geller. "Parental Experiences with Their Child's Eating Disorder Treatment Journey." *Journal of Eating Disorders* 9, no. 1 (July 2021). https://doi.org/10.1186/s40337-021-00449-x.

Even moderate dieting makes a preteen or teen . . . Golden, Neville H., Marcie Schneider, Christine Wood, Stephen R. Daniels, Steven A. Abrams, Mark R. Corkins, Sarah D. De Ferranti, et al. "Preventing Obesity and Eating Disorders in Adolescents." *Pediatrics* 138, no. 3 (September 2016). https://doi.org/10.1542/peds.2016-1649.

If your child is medically compromised . . . NEDA. "Types of Treatment." National Eating Disorders Association. Accessed February 28, 2023. https://www.nationaleatingdisorders .org/treatment/.

Family members are considered an essential part . . . Rienecke, Renee D. "Family-Based Treatment of Eating Disorders in Adolescents: Current Insights." *Adolescent Health, Medicine and Therapeutics* 8 (June 2017): 69–79. https://doi.org/10.2147/ahmt.s115775.

INDEX

ACKNOWLEDGMENTS

Nobody writes a book alone. *Kids Thrive at Every Size* wouldn't be in your hands if it weren't for the support of many.

To the families I've worked with over the years and those who follow my work: You inspire me every day with your questions, struggles, and successes. I'm grateful for your stories and challenges, as they brought humanity and humility to this book.

To Maryann Jacobsen, Heidi Schauster, Karen McGrail, Jessica Dudley, Elisabeth DiPietro, Alexia Vernon, and my husband, Jon: Your valuable feedback and kind direction undoubtedly made this a better book.

To the experts: Thank you for sharing your medical, psychology, sociology, and child-development expertise freely and generously.

To my business, nutrition, and writing colleagues: Thank you for cheering me on, supporting me through the ups and downs, and challenging me when my own self-doubt and worthiness wavered.

To my literary agent, Joelle Delbourgo: Your vision for me (and this book) exceeded mine and I am so grateful to you.

To my editor, Maisie Tivnan (and the team at Workman): Working with you has been joyful and easy. Thank you for championing my vision for *Kids Thrive at Every Size* and making it even better.

Last, to my children, Gracie, Madeline, Caroline, and Ben, and my love and life partner, Jon: I write for you and yours, always.

ABOUT THE AUTHOR

Jill Castle is one of the nation's premier childhood nutrition experts. Known for her ability to blend current research, practical application, and common sense, Jill believes that children can thrive at every size. With her paradigm-shifting, whole-child approach, she inspires parents, health-care professionals, and organizations that serve children and families to think differently about young people's health and well-being.

A sought-after speaker, advisor, and media contributor, Jill has inspired a range of audiences with her up-to-date, practical insights on childhood nutrition. She serves as a medical reviewer for Parents .com, has been featured as a guest expert on CNN, in the *Washington Post*, the *New York Times*, *Forbes*, *Newsweek*, *Time*, and many other outlets, and has consulted with schools and organizations.

Jill is the founder and CEO of The Nourished Child®, a nutrition education website and podcast for parents. She is the author of the books *Eat Like a Champion*, *Try New Food*, *The Smart Mom's Guide to Starting Solids*, and *The Smart Mom's Guide to Healthy Snacking*, and is the coauthor of *Fearless Feeding*.

Jill is the mother of four adult-ish children, and she lives in Massachusetts with her husband.